The Neuroscience of Yoga and Meditation

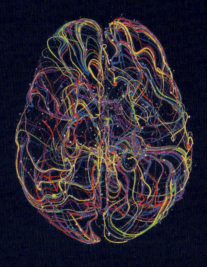

Brittany Fair, MS

Foreword by Brandt Passalacqua
Illustrated by Bruce Hogarth

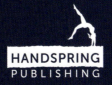

First published in Great Britain in 2023 by Handspring Publishing, an imprint of Jessica Kingsley Publishers
Part of John Murray Press

1

Copyright © Brittany Fair 2023
Foreword copyright © Brandt Passalacqua 2023

Figure 1.3 © Jeremiah Del Mar 2021, Figure 3.8 © David Heiling 2020, Figure 4.12 © Sven Mieke 2021, Figure 5.4 © Conscious Design 2020, Figure 5.6 © Thomas Evans 2020, Figures 5.9 and 8.1 © Madison Lavern 2019, Figure 5.11 © Ginny Rose Stewart 2020, Figure 5.23 © Jonny Gios, Figure 5.24 © Ant Rozetsky 2017, Figure 6.6 © Sebastian Pena Lambarri 2018, Figure 7.1 © Jared Rice 2020, Figure 8.3 © Patrick Kool 2019, Figure 9.4 © Annemiek Smegen 2020, Figure 10.9 © Frank McKenna 2016

All rights reserved. No part of this publication may be reproduced, stored in a retrieval system, or transmitted, in any form or by any means without the prior written permission of the publisher, nor be otherwise circulated in any form of binding or cover other than that in which it is published and without a similar condition being imposed on the subsequent purchaser.

Disclaimer: The information contained in this book is not intended to replace the services of trained medical professionals or to be a substitute for medical advice. The complementary therapy described in this book may not be suitable for everyone to follow. You are advised to consult a doctor before embarking on any complementary therapy programme and on any matters relating to your health, and in particular on any matters that may require diagnosis or medical attention.

A CIP catalogue record for this title is available from the British Library and the Library of Congress

ISBN 978 1 91342 643 9
eISBN 978 1 91342 644 6

Printed and bound in China by Leo Paper Products Ltd

Jessica Kingsley Publishers' policy is to use papers that are natural, renewable and recyclable products and made from wood grown in sustainable forests. The logging and manufacturing processes are expected to conform to the environmental regulations of the country of origin.

Handspring Publishing
Carmelite House
50 Victoria Embankment
London EC4Y 0DZ

www.handspringpublishing.com

John Murray Press
Part of Hodder & Stoughton Limited
An Hachette UK Company

Contents

Foreword by Brandt Passalacqua 7

Acknowledgements 10

Preface 11

1. An Introduction to Yoga and Meditation Research 13

2. The Nervous System 22

3. Anatomical Features of the Brain 36

4. The Sensory Experience of Yoga and Meditation 49

5. The Origin of Movement 67

6. The Neurophysiology of the Breath 81

7. Meditation and the Brain 95

8. Stress, Trauma and Resilience 111

9. The Effect of Yoga and Meditation on the Brain: Neurological Conditions, Chronic Pain and Addiction 131

10. Healthy Aging, Yoga and the Brain 157

Glossary 178

Subject Index 182

Author Index 187

Foreword

I had the pleasure of meeting Brittany at an annual yoga therapy research conference. I had gone there, as always, to understand more clearly why yoga practices work so well from a Western scientific perspective. I was delighted when my lunch companion told me she was a neuroscientist! As a director and lead teacher of a yoga therapy school, I had been searching for a guest teacher to enlighten my students (and myself!) on why the brain responds to movement, breath, chanting and meditation in the ways that it does.

I got into yoga therapy the way many have—through suffering. An autoimmune disease had taken root in me, and it was yoga practices that helped restore my health physically, mentally and spiritually. I became a yoga therapist, but something was still so elusive—the *why* in Western terms. How to explain *why* sitting on a cushion and chanting will help anxiety—or *why* focusing on the breath for 20 minutes each day might reduce chronic pain—or *why* moving and breathing can help someone focus in school. I have often found that clients need to understand a little bit of *why* something may work before dedicating their time to it.

The brain is a mystery to most of us. We know we have one, and we know how important it is, but most of us have no idea how it works. Yoga therapy practitioners need to be educated on the basics of brain functioning and how we can effectively influence it to our advantage.

As the years have gone by, I have found myself fielding more "*why*" questions about the efficacy of yoga practices, especially when it comes to mental health outcomes. There has been a shift away from the passive model of simply accepting that practices work, to a keen interest in the science and research of yoga therapy—and, more specifically, neuroscience and yoga. Can brain cells be regenerated? In what ways can yoga and meditation alter the brain? How can we create more healing states in the body and mind?

Over the last ten years, we've seen an explosion in yoga research, but what we haven't seen is a guidebook that distills this vast, evolving subject into an efficient, insightful lens of the effects that practices have on the nervous system and parts of the brain.

This book is just that. What is the brain? How does it interact with the body, breath and senses? What do we know and not know? As yoga practitioners, teachers and therapists, we want to wrap our minds around how yoga affects the brain, whether it be looking to compare treatment plans or simply to deepen our understanding of yoga and meditation practice.

For anyone on this quest, this book is a gift and a valuable addition to their library. Brittany has written a guide to understanding these topics, but more importantly, she gives us a chance to process such a complex subject in an accessible way.

I wish this book the success it deserves and hope it will find its place in the hands and on the bookshelves of yoga-interested people everywhere.

Brandt Passalacqua, C-IAYT, Director of Breathing Deeply Yoga Therapy

Brittany Fair, MS, RYT200, RCYT is a San Diego-based neuroscientist turned science writer, podcast host and yoga teacher. She has a passion for sharing brain-related yoga and meditation research and developed a neuroscience-based yoga workshop called NeuroFlow to provide yogis with an understanding of how meditation and yoga affect the brain. She has taught her workshop at locations across the USA including Massachusetts Institute of Technology, the Breathing Deeply Yoga Therapy School, the Bishop County Public School District as well as at numerous yoga studios. Brittany currently works as a scientific communications manager at a biological research institution and is the former president of the San Diego Science Writers Association.

The Neuroscience of Yoga and Meditation is an accessible introduction to how yoga and meditation affect the brain. Each chapter guides the reader through the latest yoga and meditation research. The book also explores the current limitations in studying these practices and offers tools for interpreting scientific literature. The chapters provide examples of yoga routines and meditations that can be adapted for different populations. Although the book does not contain an exhaustive explanation of all medical conditions or diseases, it was designed to inform the yoga teacher sufficiently to work with a variety of students.

Acknowledgements

Accepting this book deal while pregnant with twins was one of the wildest things I've ever done. I wrote most of this book during my first year of motherhood with two boys who didn't sleep through the night, while balancing a full-time job. None of this would have been possible without my incredible husband Dustin. He has edited every chapter of this book multiple times, wrangled twins, and let me sleep so that I could write some more. He is my hero, and I have promised him that I will not accept another book deal while pregnant.

I am also grateful for my mother Vickie and father David for always being supportive of my dreams. They have combed through this book, identifying grammatical errors and inconsistencies time and time again.

Thank you to my wonderful yoga friends Phil and Ashley for reading through chapters and providing feedback. Your thoughtful comments helped shape this book for the better. Finally, thank you to all of those who helped me to get here: Caitlin, Sarah, Leah, Cheryl, Ally and many more. Your love and support made this dream a reality.

Preface

I was first introduced to yoga in college when I signed up for a Power Yoga course on a whim. While I considered myself an athlete and physically fit, I found that I did not have the stamina for even some of the simplest poses. But it wasn't until graduate school that my practice started to expand.

As a neuroscience graduate student at the The Robert Larner College of Medicine at The University of Vermont, I spent my mornings in the anatomy lab, mastering the use of a scalpel to meticulously dissect a human cadaver. My afternoons and evenings were spent in the library, trying to cram as much information into my brain as humanly possible. My world was restricted to these activities. I had no work–life balance.

In my second year of graduate school, this lifestyle began to catch up with me. Studying, teaching and pursuing my research led to elevated levels of stress and anxiety. I returned to yoga looking for relief and soon it became a passion. I decided to sign up for a 200hr yoga teacher training at a local yoga school called Sangha Studio in Burlington, Vermont. This is where my journey into contemplative practices began.

Before attending training, I assumed yoga was synonymous with movement, but I quickly learned about the anatomy, history, spirituality, breath and other aspects that were equally (if not more) important to a practice. I also started a regular meditation practice and attended a meditation retreat at the Shambhala Buddhist retreat center Karmê Chöling. Meditating every day was one of the hardest things I had ever done. For hours we knelt in silence, acknowledging our thoughts and letting them gently float away. It was emotionally and mentally taxing, but it was also freeing. I felt more clarity than I had felt in a long time.

In graduate school, I had been studying the neural basis of personality, but understanding the science behind yoga and meditation was my true dream. I was fascinated by how the brain could be altered by something seemingly as simple as the breath. My deep interest in the science of yoga and meditation led me to become a regular contributor to Yoga Research & Beyond, an online research library filled with easy-to-read reviews of academic articles.

I also developed a yoga workshop called NeuroFlow that explores the latest yoga and meditation research findings. My first workshop was held at Sangha Studio where I completed my teacher training. To make sure the workshop was as interactive as possible, I decided I wanted to bring along a real brain. Finding a brain on short notice was surprisingly easy in Vermont, as a local sheep farmer had had a sheep pass away the night before. It took some ingenuity to carefully extract the brain without damaging any of the delicate tissue. But at my workshop the next day, I was able to point out brain anatomy on this small, perfect specimen of a sheep brain. That brain brought the workshop to life.

Although this book does not include a real sheep's brain, I hope the book illustrates some of the many exciting neuroscience topics that are related to yoga and meditation. This book is not an encyclopedia of every available study, but rather it includes material that will hopefully spark curiosity about how yoga and meditation can affect our bodies, change our minds and alter the way our cells function.

My intention is that this book will help demystify the brain and share why yoga and meditation lead to so many mental and physical health benefits. Although the research in this field is relatively new, it is an exciting time to witness the rapid increase in studies and rigor that is occurring across the field. I believe that the evidence supporting how yoga and meditation benefit the brain will continue to grow in the years to come.

I am excited to share this project with you. I hope you enjoy it.

Sincerely,

Brittany Fair, MS, 2023

CHAPTER 1

An Introduction to Yoga and Meditation Research

The practice of yoga and meditation has increasingly become the focus of scientific research. Studies aim to validate their health benefits. Do yoga and meditation effectively reduce stress? Offer an alternative approach to ameliorate certain conditions and diseases? Help with sleep and mood disorders? It can be challenging to sort through and understand the science behind yoga and meditation studies. Many have been questioned due to low quality. They are often based on small sample sizes and rely on self-reported questionnaires instead of biological data. In this chapter, we will review important considerations for evaluating key studies and discuss what to look for when assessing the results.

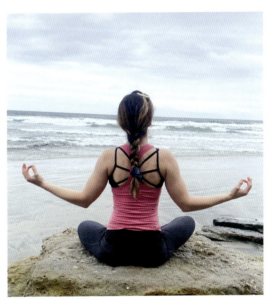

Figure 1.1 Meditation by the sea to promote relaxation.

INTRODUCTION

For centuries, practitioners of yoga and meditation have reported feeling calm, refreshed and centered (Figure 1.1). Archeologists and historians have dated the original practice of meditation to sometime around 1500 BCE (Freeman et al., 2019). Yet, no one knows the exact origins of meditative practices. Only recently have scientists begun to understand how these contemplative practices impact the brain.

The human brain is malleable. New research suggests that regularly practicing yoga and meditation can alter the brain in a multitude of ways. For example, regions of the brain involved in empathy can be activated and strengthened by practicing loving-kindness meditation (Lutz et al., 2008). These exercises can change neural pathways that allow practitioners to be more kind, compassionate humans as well as to live longer, healthier lives.

Brain imaging is not required to understand that yoga and meditation have a positive impact on health. These practices have been widely reported to provide physical and mental health benefits, leading to an influx of practitioners in the Western world. In fact, more than 32 million people currently practice yoga in the United States, though they are not representative of the general population (Zhang *et al.*, 2021). The 2017 National Health Interview Survey, one of the largest and most comprehensive health surveys in the United States, showed that women are more than twice as likely to practice yoga as men, and yoga is most popular among non-Hispanic white adults aged 18–44 (Clarke *et al.*, 2018; CDC, 2018; NCCIH, 2020).

The rapidly growing interest in contemplative practices has also driven curiosity in the research world to understand *how* these practices are affecting the mind and body. In the last ten years, the fields of yoga and meditation research have exploded. Publications have increased exponentially, from virtually nothing in 1950 to now thousands of manuscripts related to these practices. The rigor of these scientific studies is also improving, which will help bring further legitimacy to the fields. Researchers from major universities and hospitals are now exploring how yoga and meditation impact health, including changes to the brain.

DEFINING YOGA

Yoga originated in India as a spiritual practice. One of the first yogic texts is the *Yoga Sutras of Patanjali*, which dates to the early centuries CE (Schmalzl, Powers and Henje Blom, 2015). The word "yoga" is translated from the Sanskrit word "yug" or "yuj," which means "union" or "method of spiritual union" (Van Aalst *et al.*, 2020). The goal of traditional practice was to achieve a state in which there is balance between the mind and body, as well as between the individual and the greater good.

Today, yoga is often thought of as a meditative movement practice. The growth in practitioners and interest has led to a plethora of yoga styles in the Western world, including Vinyasa, Hatha, Iyengar, restorative and many more. Some yoga styles, such as Power Yoga, emphasize physical postures, while others focus more on meditation and breathing techniques. Yoga in the West is generally thought of as a physical practice, whereas Eastern yoga tends to emphasize the breath and meditative practices (Schmalzl, Powers and Henje Blom, 2015).

The wide range of practices that can be called yoga can make it difficult to tell what is being examined in a research study. The type of yoga or meditation used in these studies is often unclear or not explicitly stated, obscuring conclusions about different styles of yoga. Instead, conclusions are usually based on the all-encompassing term "yoga" or "meditation," and studies seek to understand how these general practices reduce stress, improve health and increase self-regulation.

Recently, scientists recognized the need for a clearer definition of yoga to use in research studies, and the National Institutes of Health funded the creation of a questionnaire that could be used in studies moving forward. The Essential Properties of Yoga Questionnaire, created by scientists at the University of California, San Diego, contains 62 questions about 14 dimensions of a yoga class, including components such as compassion, breathwork, body awareness, yoga philosophy and more (Park *et al.*, 2018). Scientists can now use this questionnaire to better quantify the type of yoga intervention they are using in their studies (Figure 1.2).

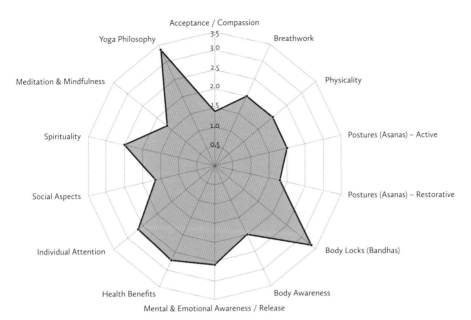

Figure 1.2 The Essential Properties of Yoga Questionnaire: schematic showing the 14 dimensions.
Source: Image courtesy of Erik Groessl from the University of California, San Diego. From: https://epyqview.ucsd.edu

CHALLENGES IN YOGA AND MEDITATION RESEARCH

Many yoga and meditation studies suffer from a small sample size (typically fewer than 20 people) and a homogeneous group of participants (usually Caucasian middle-aged women), so it is difficult to say if the results would hold true for every person. Many studies are also conducted using self-reported questionnaires, a method that can be prone to bias. Despite these limitations, yoga and meditation research is open to so many possibilities with the advancement of neuroimaging technologies and molecular tools. As the field progresses, the rigor of research will also improve.

What is scientific evidence?
Scientific evidence is derived from a well-controlled study that statistically either supports or counters a hypothesis or theory.

What is a variable?
A **variable** is any factor that a scientist is changing or measuring in some way. In yoga and meditation research, many different variables can be measured, such as the type or quantity of yoga practice, stress hormones and mental health measures.

COMMON RESEARCH METHODOLOGIES AND STUDY DESIGN

Not all research studies are created equal. There are many different types of scientific evidence that can be presented as research. For example, a scientist may write a perspective or an editorial in a research journal, or a team of researchers may conduct a randomized control trial. What are the major differences between these types of approaches, and why do they matter?

Perspectives and editorials rely on someone's opinion instead of the data from a specific study. Although they are not technically considered scientific evidence, they can be helpful for inspiring better-designed studies in the future.

Case studies are rarely used in yoga research but are common in medical research. A case study is an in-depth analysis of a single person, group or situation. It may provide evidence about one of these three specific things, but the sample size is small (usually one person), and it is impossible to deduce if the results would hold broadly true for other people, groups or situations. The results are retrospective and not predictive.

Cohort studies are common in yoga and meditation research. A researcher tracks a group of participants longitudinally, over time, typically before and after an intervention. For instance, a scientist may test participants' hormone levels before and after practicing yoga to better understand the impact of yoga on hormone levels. Cohort studies can also last for extended periods of time. The Framingham Study investigating risk factors for heart disease is one of the largest and longest consecutively running cohort studies ever conducted, dating back to 1948.

Randomized control trials are the gold standard in research. Participants in a randomized control trial are randomly assigned to either the experimental group (the group receiving the intervention, i.e., practicing yoga or meditation) or the control group. These groups are then compared. Randomized control trials are common in medical research and often conducted as a double-blind study where neither the researcher nor the participant knows if they are receiving the drug or the placebo. Blind or double-blind studies are nearly impossible to conduct in yoga research because a study participant can easily guess if they're in the experimental group (practicing yoga) or the control group (not practicing yoga).

Thus, there is room for bias, and bias should be considered when examining the results.

Reviews combine evidence from multiple research studies. A systematic review answers a defined research question using clear and predetermined eligibility criteria for including certain studies. Review articles often contain meta-analyses, which use statistics to summarize the results of studies. The scientist conducting a review is not carrying out a physical study, but rather analyzing previous studies to answer a research question. This method is a powerful tool for understanding the larger picture as it considers much more data than a single study (Ahn and Kang, 2018).

What type of paper should I read first?

If you're new to the subject area, a review article is an excellent place to start. It's like choosing to watch a movie about African animals, instead of a documentary that only focuses on giraffes. Now, if you're really into giraffes then go for it! But otherwise, it can be nice to gain some background information before diving in deep.

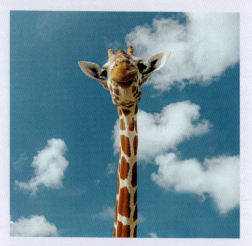

Figure 1.3 A giraffe in Coron, Palawan, Philippines.
Source: Jeremiah Del Mar on Unsplash.

QUANTITATIVE VS. QUALITATIVE METHODS

Both quantitative and qualitative methods can be used to examine how yoga and meditation affect the body and mind. While quantitative data is number driven, qualitative data is descriptive and conceptual.

Quantitative data refers to information that can be counted or measured. In yoga research, scientists may measure how much a person's blood pressure changes from the yoga intervention. The change in blood pressure is a number that can be easily analyzed and compared. Most data collected in the field of biological science is quantitative data.

Qualitative data is descriptive in nature and represented with language, instead of numbers. Some scientists use qualitative data to examine things that are hard to quantify, such as the "why" or the "how." For example, a researcher might use an in-depth interview to ask *how* the yoga intervention made the participants feel more involved in their community.

So, what are some advantages and disadvantages of each strategy? Quantitative data can be analyzed and replicated by another group of scientists to see if they get the same result. If multiple studies find the same results, then that builds evidence that the result is accurate. Quantitative data doesn't always tell the full story; numbers and measurements cannot easily capture things like feelings and emotions. Broader relationships can be missed or overlooked.

Qualitative data, on the other hand, offers rich, descriptive insights into relationships and can be great for exploratory purposes. Because qualitative observations require interpretation, they can be difficult to analyze without bias. Quantitative data is generally preferred across neuroscience research because it is structured and concrete, although some scientists believe that the best designed studies will have both types of data represented.

THE IMPORTANCE OF SAMPLE SIZE

Sample size is the number of subjects chosen for an experiment. It is one of the most important factors in designing a research study because it can inherently impact the results. Small samples can negatively affect the validity of a study because the results often cannot be generalized to another group or population. Conversely, extremely large samples can transform small variations into statistically significant differences and amplify study bias (Faber and Fonseca, 2014; Kaplan, Chambers and Glasgow, 2014). Therefore, the sample size of a study should be considered as important as any other variable.

> **What is validity?**
> **External validity** is the ability to generalize results from a study to a broader population outside of the study. For instance, if a researcher found that practicing Yin yoga three times a week decreased cortisol levels, then another scientist should be able to replicate the study with another group of people and find the same results. This would mean that the study had a high external validity.
>
> **Internal validity** is when the results from one group within the study can be generalized to another group within the study. It demonstrates that the methods can reliably produce the same results, and the results are not explained by other factors. A well-designed study will have high internal validity because the findings are consistent across groups.

Yoga and meditation studies tend to suffer from small, homogeneous sample sizes. Typically, samples range from around 12 to 25 participants, which is considered small for research involving human subjects. It can be nearly impossible to draw results that are meaningful with so few subjects. Let's say that scientists found that 15 middle-aged women had lower levels of stress after doing a headstand for two minutes – would the same results be true for elderly men? A larger study with a more diverse population would need to be conducted to find out. If 100 individuals of varying ethnicities, age and overall health status found that two minutes of headstand improved their stress levels, it could mean that headstand helps to reduce stress. The results would be even more convincing if they were replicated in an additional study using even more participants.

THE DIFFERENCE BETWEEN CAUSATION AND CORRELATION

"Causation" and "correlation" are common terms in the research world, but what do they really mean?

Causation occurs when one variable is directly related to or *causes* the second variable. In science, causation is extremely difficult to prove. In yoga research, studies will often make claims like "stretching causes increased flexibility." Without a mechanistic understanding of stretching and flexibility, it is actually hard to prove that one directly causes the other. Instead, stretching and flexibility are strongly related or correlated. If a scientist believed that stretching led to an increase in flexibility and then dissected the limb to understand exactly what changed internally to cause this strong relationship, then causality could be proven. Alas, we are not going to cut open the limbs of our yoga subjects to prove without a doubt that stretching causes increased flexibility. We'll just have to rely on common sense and a mechanistic understanding of stretching and flexibility in animals to reason that the causality in this relationship is highly likely.

> **What is statistical significance?**
> **Statistical significance** is a measure of confidence that two variables are related in some way and that the result is not due to chance.

Correlation is a measure of how strongly two variables are related, but one may not cause the other. Almost all yoga and meditation studies represent correlations, not causations. Two variables can be correlated with one another, but it does not mean that one variable causes the other. Sometimes variables can be highly correlated but not be causally related at all, or they could have a common cause.

When the two variables are highly correlated but not causally related, they are called spurious correlations. For instance, the number of letters in the winning word of the Scripps National Spelling Bee is correlated with the number of people killed each year by venomous spiders (Vigen, 2022). Clearly, the number of letters of the winning word is not *causing* people to die from venomous spiders. This correlation is nothing more than a coincidence (Figure 1.4).

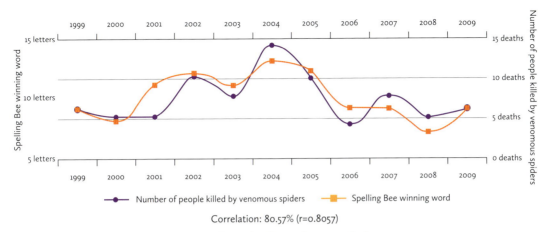

Figure 1.4 Example of a spurious correlation.

Source: Image courtesy of Tyler Vigen, CC BY 4.0. From: http://www.tylervigen.com/spurious-correlations

HOW TO DISSECT A RESEARCH STUDY

There are many ways to approach a research study. A majority of scientists polled on Twitter preferred to start with the results section, likely because they already know the subject matter well and want to get to the key findings as fast as possible. For readers unfamiliar with a given field of research, it may be easiest to start with the introduction section to understand the background of the subject matter, then move on to the rest of the study.

- **Introduction:** The introduction is where the researchers review previous findings, point out what is lacking in the field and say how their study fills an important gap. Someone with little knowledge of the subject could read the introduction to get a basic idea of what the study was about.
- **Methods:** In this section, researchers describe the experiments that were used to answer a research question and explain how results were analyzed. The methods include information about factors such as: 1) how many people participated in the study, 2) the demographics of these people, 3) information about a comparison group or comparison condition, and 4) the attrition rate (i.e., did people drop out).
- **Results:** As the name suggests, the results section presents key findings of a published article. It typically contains a lot of data and numbers without much interpretation.
- **Discussion:** Here, the researchers explore the meaning of their results as well as the implications of their work. Authors often explain how their study fits in to the greater context of the scientific literature and point to opportunities for future studies.

OTHER FACTORS TO CONSIDER

There are many additional reported benefits to practicing yoga and meditation that are often unaccounted for in research studies. For example, contemplative practices often allow individuals to meet a community of like-minded people. This can lead to lifestyle changes, such as exercising more and eating healthier foods, thereby increasing the benefits of yoga and meditation, creating a positive feedback loop.

There is also the possibility of participant bias. Many people who are willing to participate in a study about yoga or meditation may already be inclined towards a healthy lifestyle. Thus, their baseline health may be different than that of a participant who is trying yoga or meditation for the first time.

These variables are often overlooked in research studies as they are difficult to measure. Scientists tend to focus on the immediate and direct impact of yoga or meditation on mental and physical health. Thus, the conclusions drawn are an incomplete picture of the full effects of contemplative practices on health.

Many of the studies discussed in this book are well designed, but these factors are something that you, as the reader, should consider when understanding the greater context of this research.

> **Main takeaways**
> - Yoga is often defined as a meditative movement practice in research.
> - There are many different types of scientific evidence that can be presented as research, including cohort studies, randomized control trials, reviews and many more.
> - Quantitative data refers to information that can be counted or measured, whereas qualitative data is descriptive in nature and represented with language.
> - Almost all yoga and meditation studies represent correlations, not causations.
> - Yoga and meditation research will undoubtedly become more rigorous as the field advances.

REFERENCES

Ahn, E.J., & Kang, H., 2018. Introduction to systematic review and meta-analysis. *Korean Journal of Anesthesiology*, 71(2), pp.103-112.

Centers for Disease Control and Prevention (CDC), 2018. Use of yoga and meditation becoming more popular in U.S. Available at: https://www.cdc.gov/nchs/pressroom/nchs_press_releases/2018/201811_Yoga_Meditation.htm

Clarke, T.C., Barnes, P.M., Black, L.I., Stussman, B.J., & Nahin, R.L., 2018. Use of yoga, meditation, and chiropractors among U.S. adults aged 18 and over. NCHS Data Brief, no. 325. Hyattsville, MD: National Center for Health Statistics. Available at: https://www.cdc.gov/nchs/data/databriefs/db325-h.pdf

Faber, J., & Fonseca, L.M., 2014. How sample size influences research outcomes. *Dental Press Journal of Orthodontics*, 19(4), pp.27-29.

Freeman Jr., R.C., Sukuan, N., Tota, N.M., Bell, S.M., Harris, A.G., & Wang, H.L., 2019. Promoting spiritual healing by stress reduction through meditation for employees at a Veterans Hospital: a CDC framework-based program evaluation. *Workplace Health & Safety*, 68(4), pp.161-170.

Kaplan, R.M., Chambers, D.A., & Glasgow, R.E., 2014. Big Data and large sample size: a cautionary note on the potential for bias. *Clinical and Translational Science*, 7(4), pp.342-346.

Lutz, A., Brefczynski-Lewis, J., Johnstone, T., & Davidson, R.J., 2008. Regulation of the neural circuitry of emotion by compassion meditation: effects of meditative expertise. *PLoS ONE*, 3(3), e1897.

National Center for Complementary and Integrative Health (NCCIH), 2020. *Yoga for Health*. Available at: https://files.nccih.nih.gov/s3fs-public/Yoga-eBook-2020_06_FINAL_508.pdf

Park, C.L., Elwy, A.R., Maiya, M., Sarkin, A.J., et al., 2018. The Essential Properties of Yoga Questionnaire (EPYQ): psychometric properties. *International Journal of Yoga Therapy*, 28(1), pp.23-38.

Schmalzl, L., Powers, C., & Henje Blom, E., 2015. Neurophysiological and neurocognitive mechanisms underlying the effects of yoga-based practices: towards a comprehensive theoretical framework. *Frontiers in Human Neuroscience*, 9, p.235.

van Aalst, J., Ceccarini, J., Demyttenaere, K., Sunaert, S., & Van Laere, K., 2020. What has neuroimaging taught us on the neurobiology of yoga? A review. *Frontiers in Integrative Neuroscience*, 14, p.34.

Vigen, T., 2022. *Spurious Correlations*. Available at: http://www.tylervigen.com/spurious-correlations

Zhang, Y., Lauche, R., Cramer, H., Munk, N., & Dennis, J.A., 2021. Increasing trend of yoga practice among U.S. adults from 2002 to 2017. *Journal of Alternative Complementary Medicine*, 27(9), pp. 778–785.

The Nervous System

Yoga and meditation impact the nervous system, the complex web of neurons and nerves that connect every organ and tissue in the body. This chapter will dive into the basics of the nervous system to explore how these practices can influence the sympathetic nervous system and the parasympathetic nervous system through breathing, movement and stress reduction. It will also cover the basic anatomy of brain cells and the molecules they use for communication called neurotransmitters.

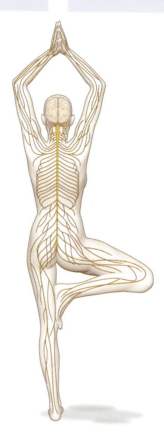

Figure 2.1 The nervous system with the brain, spinal cord and nerves.

INTRODUCTION

The nervous system (Figure 2.1) has two main branches: the **central nervous system** (CNS) and the **peripheral nervous system** (PNS). The CNS includes the brain and the spinal cord, while the PNS consists of the neurons and nerves that stretch throughout the body (Figure 2.2).

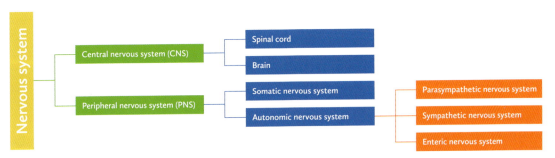

Figure 2.2 The organization of the nervous system.

The PNS can be further broken down into two main subsystems: the somatic and the autonomic nervous systems. The **somatic nervous system** carries information about voluntary movement, while the **autonomic nervous system** relays information about automatic or involuntary responses. The autonomic nervous system is the body's autopilot and can function without conscious thought. Some of the functions include regulating the breath, heart rate and digestion (Figure 2.3).

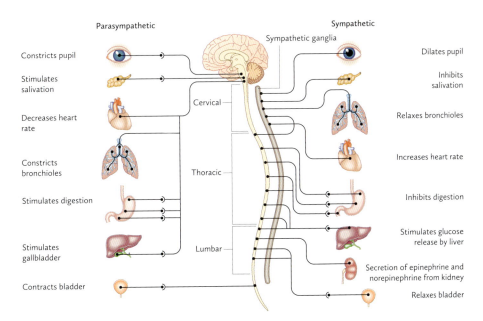

Figure 2.3 The differences between the parasympathetic and sympathetic nervous systems. Each nervous system acts in different ways to regulate the body.

Yoga and meditation research often focuses on the autonomic nervous system, which includes the sympathetic, parasympathetic and enteric nervous systems. The **sympathetic nervous system** is activated during periods of stress as well as rigorous activity. It is commonly thought to control the fight, flight or freeze response when faced with danger. For instance, when encountering a lion, the natural response might be to fight the lion, run away from the lion, or freeze to not attract attention. Yoga, meditation and other relaxation techniques have been shown to decrease sympathetic nervous system activity, which can enhance decision making in the face of immediate stressors (Vempati and Telles, 2002; Starcke and Brand, 2012).

In contrast, the **parasympathetic nervous system** controls the relaxation response. It helps the body calm down, relax the muscles and digest food. It also becomes more active during periods of gentle movement, breathing exercises and meditation (Anasuya, Deepak and Jaryal, 2021). The sympathetic nervous system and the parasympathetic nervous system work together to maintain balance, or homeostasis, in the body.

Restorative yoga is an accessible tool for activating the parasympathetic nervous system and downregulating the sympathetic nervous system (Figure 2.4). It can reduce stress and slow heart rate while improving emotional state, metabolism and fatigue (Danhauer *et al.*, 2009; Kanaya *et al.*, 2014; Leong, 2019). The technique was built on the teachings of B.K.S. Iyengar and popularized in the 1970s by Judith Lasater, who studied under Iyengar (Leong, 2019). Restorative yoga involves holding comfortable yoga postures for longer periods of time supported by props, such as blocks, bolsters and blankets. The focus is placed on the breath or music to promote a deep state of relaxation. This slow, supported practice is ideal for those experiencing stress who seek to restore and heal the body.

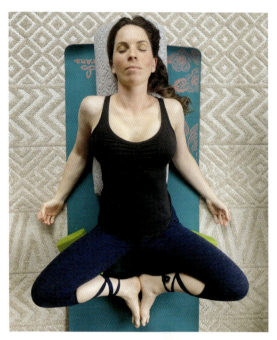

Figure 2.4 Reclined bound angle pose using a bolster and two blocks.

EXAMPLE RESTORATIVE YOGA CLASS TO PROMOTE RELAXATION

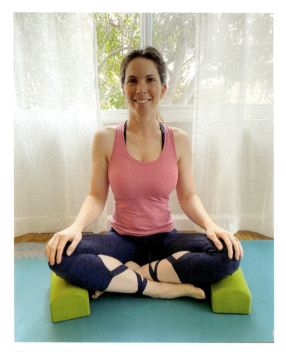

Figure 2.5 Supported easy pose with two blocks.

THE NERVOUS SYSTEM   25

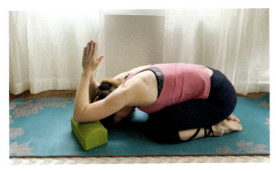

Figure 2.6 Child's pose variation with two blocks.

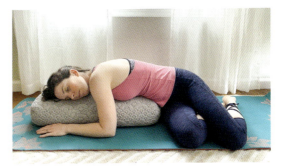

Figure 2.10 Supported spinal twist with bolster.

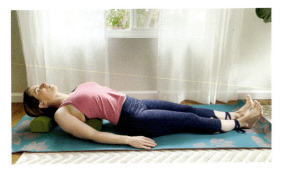

Figure 2.7 Supported fish pose with two blocks.

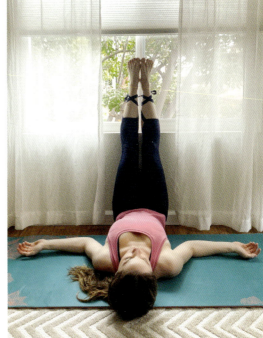

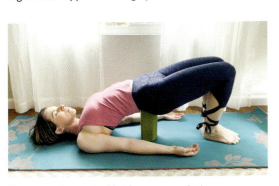

Figure 2.8 Supported bridge pose variation.

Figure 2.11 Legs-up-the-wall pose.

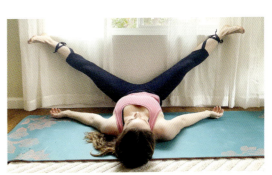

Figure 2.9 Supported bridge pose variation.

Figure 2.12 Legs-up-the-wall pose variation.

The vagus nerve

The vagus nerve, also known as the 10th cranial nerve (CN X), is the main nerve of the parasympathetic nervous system. It extends from the brainstem to the colon (also called the large intestine) and helps control the heart, lungs and digestive tract. It is considered a key link between the gut and the brain.

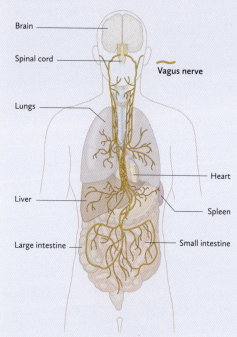

Figure 2.13 Vagus nerve anatomy.

Contemplative practices stimulate the vagus nerve, promoting relaxation through increased activity of the parasympathetic nervous system. The parasympathetic nervous system slows the stress response to help reduce inflammation and stress hormones in the body (Streeter *et al.*, 2012; McCall, 2013).

Vagus nerve stimulation can also be conducted in the clinic using a device that generates electrical impulses. Vagus nerve stimulation is currently approved by the US Food and Drug Administration (FDA) to treat epilepsy and depression. It is also being studied to treat other conditions, including traumatic brain injury, rheumatoid arthritis and stroke, due to its anti-inflammatory effects (Johnson and Wilson, 2018).

Fun fact

The gut produces nearly 95 percent of the serotonin made in the body (Kim and Camilleri, 2000). Serotonin is a neurotransmitter or signaling molecule that helps regulate mood, sleep and appetite. The other five percent is produced in a small region of the brainstem called the raphe nuclei (Berger, Gray and Roth, 2009).

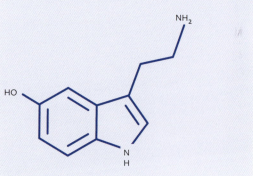

Figure 2.14 Serotonin molecule.

The third autonomic nervous system is the **enteric nervous system**. It oversees most of the digestive functions, such as movements of the gastrointestinal tract, and regulates the secretion of digestive fluids and hormones. It also stimulates the immune system (Fleming *et al.*, 2020). The enteric nervous system can send and receive signals from the CNS as well as function independently.

It is estimated that the enteric nervous system contains between 400 and 600 million neurons and produces most of the body's serotonin, a neurotransmitter that affects brain activity and is involved in mood (Fleming et al., 2020). Thus, the enteric nervous system is also called the "second brain."

Research on the enteric nervous system has shown that an altered gut microbiota can affect mental health and is related to neurodegenerative diseases, such as Alzheimer's and Parkinson's (Rao and Gershon, 2016; Rieder et al., 2017; Fleming et al., 2020). Conversely, contemplative practices such as yoga and meditation have been shown to improve the gut microbiome and symptoms of gut-associated disorders, such as irritable bowel syndrome (Tavassoli, 2009; Asare, Störsrud and Simrén, 2012; Jia et al., 2020). Irritable bowel syndrome is linked to stress and inflammation, and these practices may reduce these factors to positively impact and heal the gut.

Main takeaways
- The nervous system consists of two main systems: the central nervous system and the peripheral nervous system.
- The sympathetic and the parasympathetic nervous systems work together to maintain balance in the body.
- Relaxation practices can reduce sympathetic activity and increase parasympathetic activity.
- Both yoga and meditation promote gut health by reducing stress and inflammation, which improves the gut microbiome.

AN INTRODUCTION TO THE BRAIN

The commander of the central nervous system is the brain. It gives rise to conscious thought, movement and emotions. Despite its important role, a human brain weighs only three pounds. That's about the same weight as a small bag of potatoes. The brain's densely packed tissue contains approximately 86 billion specialized brain cells called neurons, and it has an additional 85 billion non-neuronal support cells called glia (Herculano-Houzel, 2012).

Each of those 86 billion neurons has thousands of connections with other cells (Hawkins and Ahmad, 2016). These connections are called synapses and they allow one neuron to send a signal to another, typically in a burst of chemicals called neurotransmitters. Together, neurons form over 100 trillion connections throughout the brain (Parhi and Unnikrishnan, 2020).

Neurons are a special class of cells that transmit information throughout the body and brain. Like other cells, neurons have a cell body (called the soma) with a nucleus inside surrounded by a cellular membrane. Near the soma, neurons have protrusions called dendrites that branch out and connect to other cells and neurons (Figure 2.15). These dendrites receive chemical signals from hundreds or even thousands of other cells.

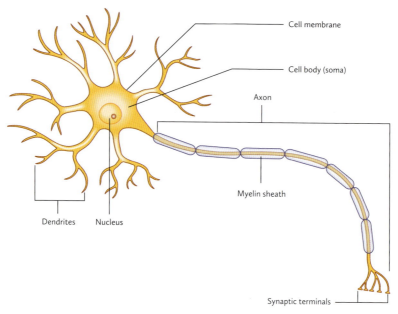

Figure 2.15 The anatomy of a neuron.

On the other side of the cell body is a long, thin axon. The axon conducts electrical signals down to the synaptic terminals where one neuron connects to the dendrites of another neuron.

How do neurons communicate?

Neurons control signaling in the brain by communicating with one another through neurotransmitters. Neurotransmitters can be excitatory or inhibitory (see Neurotransmitters 101), which can either promote or inhibit an action potential in the receiving neuron.

Every neuron in the brain is constantly receiving signals. When the excitatory inputs become greater than the inhibitory inputs, an action potential occurs. An action potential is an electrical signal that is sent down the neuron's axon towards another neuron. When the action potential reaches the small gap between the two neurons, called the synaptic cleft, it causes neurotransmitters to be released in the gap (Figure 2.16). Neurotransmitters bind to receptor sites on the receiving neuron's dendrites. The first neuron then takes back some of its neurotransmitter in a process called reuptake so the cell signaling can occur again.

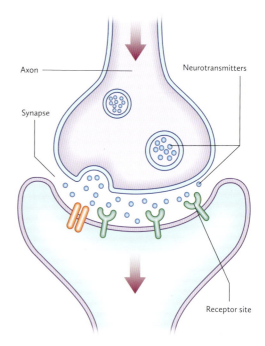

Figure 2.16 The synapse and release of neurotransmitters.

Neurotransmitters 101

Neurotransmitters are molecules that carry a signal from one neuron to another. There are thought to be over 100 different types of neurotransmitters (Si and Song, 2018). Some common neurotransmitters are acetylcholine, dopamine, norepinephrine, serotonin, gamma-aminobutyric acid (GABA) and glutamate.

- **Acetylcholine** is involved in a variety of functions, including contracting muscles, arousal, attention, memory, learning and recall.
- **Dopamine** is the main neurotransmitter used in the reward system of the brain. When a person anticipates a reward, such as winning a prize, dopamine levels increase in the brain. Through these brain pathways, it is also linked with addiction and substance abuse. Dopamine is also an important molecule for movement. Dopamine pathways do not function properly in conditions like Parkinson's disease (Segura-Aguilar et al., 2014).
- **Norepinephrine** is used in the brain and body to prepare for arousal during exercise, stress and danger. It constricts blood vessels to raise blood pressure. Additionally, it can trigger anxiety, may be involved in depression, and plays a role in motivation and reward (Goddard et al., 2010; España, Schmeichel and Berridge, 2016).
- **Serotonin** helps regulate mood, sleep and appetite. It is also thought to inhibit pain (Bardin, 2011). Although some of this neurotransmitter is created in the brain, roughly 95 percent of serotonin in the body is created in the gut.
- **Gamma-aminobutyric acid** (GABA) is an inhibitory neurotransmitter and reduces the amount of communication between neurons in the brain. Overall, GABA decreases the activity of the nervous system. It is likely dysregulated in conditions such as anxiety and depression (Kalueff and Nutt, 2007).
- **Glutamate** is the main excitatory neurotransmitter in the brain, and it may play a role in bipolar disorder and schizophrenia (Goff and Coyle, 2001). Medications that contain lithium carbonate provide mood stabilizing effects and might stabilize glutamate levels in the brain.

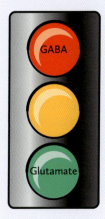

Figure 2.17 GABA and glutamate regulate the action potentials of neurons. Since GABA is an inhibitory neurotransmitter, it stops action potentials. Glutamate is an excitatory neurotransmitter and can start an action potential or keep an action potential moving.

Main takeaways

- The human brain weighs about three pounds and contains 86 billion neurons.
- Neurons communicate with one another through electrical events called action potentials that lead to the

release of chemical messengers called neurotransmitters.
- Neurotransmitters allow neurons to communicate with one another.

Other cells in the brain

There are many other types of cells in the brain besides neurons. In fact, nearly half the cells in the brain are cells called glia. Unlike neurons, glia do not fire action potentials, which has led neuroscientists to overlook glia and their role in the brain for a very long time (Allen and Barres, 2009). Glia are now recognized for their many diverse roles in the brain, including influencing how neurons communicate and providing nutrients for growth (Temburni and Jacob, 2001). Three main types of glia are microglia, oligodendrocytes and astrocytes (Figure 2.18).

Microglia are the brain's immune cells, and they monitor the brain's environment for any intruders, such as bacteria and viruses. Microglia also act as the brain's garbagemen, cleaning up debris, and as the brain's gardener, pruning back unnecessary neuronal connections. In certain brain disorders such as Alzheimer's disease, the brain's microglia may become hyperactive, leading to inflammation and the deposit of toxic proteins known as amyloid plaques and neurofibrillary tangles (Hansen, Hanson and Sheng, 2017).

Oligodendrocytes help to insulate the axons of neurons in the brain that travel long distances by wrapping them in a protective myelin sheath. The myelin sheath acts as insulation to help neurons transmit their signals as fast as possible. Oligodendrocytes are the brain's electricians. They wrap axons in insulation like how an electrician would wrap a power cable.

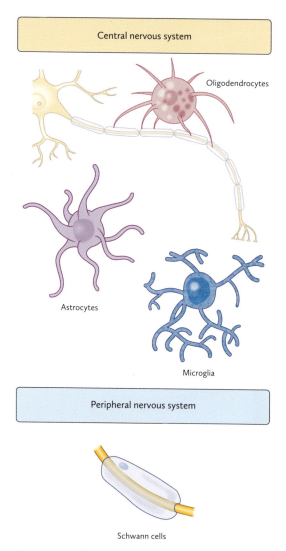

Figure 2.18 Different types of glia in the brain.
Source: Blausen.com staff (2014), CC BY 3.0 via Commons. From: https://qbi.uq.edu.au/brain-basics/brain/brain-physiology/types-glia

Fun fact

Some animals, such as squid, do not have myelin. Instead, they have a giant axon about the diameter of a pencil, which is roughly 1,000 times wider than a typical human axon (Coles, 2015). The wider diameter helps them transmit signals faster since they lack myelin.

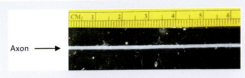

Figure 2.19 A giant axon from the squid *Dosidicus gigas*.
Source: Mathur et al., Creative Commons. From: http://nerve.bsd.uchicago.edu/nervejs/NERVEhelp.html

During the 1950s, neuroscientists Alan Hodgkin and Andrew Huxley wanted to study neurons, but they were limited by technology. So, they used squid to learn more about these hard-to-visualize cells. Since the squid axons were so large, they were easier to study, and the scientists could examine how action potentials worked for the first time (Hodgkin, Huxley and Katz, 1952). Hodgkin and Huxley were later awarded the Nobel Prize in Physiology or Medicine in 1963 for their discovery.

Astrocytes are star-shaped cells that shuttle nutrients to neurons and aid in neuron-to-neuron communication. Astrocytes regulate the amount of neurotransmitter around the neuron's synapse (Newman, 2003). There is ongoing research into how astrocytes help neurons communicate.

There are many other important types of glial cells. For instance, **Schwann cells** are similar to oligodendrocytes, but are found in the peripheral nervous system instead of the central nervous system. There are also **epithelial cells** that help keep invaders from getting into the brain's blood system, and **ependymal cells** that produce cerebrospinal fluid, among others.

THE SPINAL CORD

The central nervous system also includes the **spinal cord** (Figure 2.20), a bundle of nerves that extends about 46 centimeters (18 inches) from the brain to the lumbar vertebrae in the lower back (Boonpirak and Apinhasmit, 1994).

Although the spinal cord is only around one centimeter in diameter, it contains roughly one billion neurons (Saritas *et al.*, 2008; Nagel *et al.*, 2017). Thus, the spinal cord acts like an information highway carrying signals between the brain and the body. The spinal cord is involved in both voluntary and involuntary movement. For example, the spinal cord transmits signals from the brain to the muscles of the legs to enable movement, and it innervates the lungs independently of the brain for breathing.

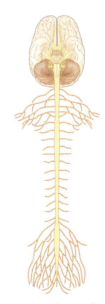

Figure 2.20 The spinal cord extending from the base of the brain.

The spinal cord can also send signals directly to the muscles without the brain during reflexive movements. Reflexes are automatic, involuntary responses to sensory inputs, like accidentally touching a hot pan. The hand is automatically pulled back in a withdrawal reflex to avoid a burn. This action bypasses the brain and is processed solely by the spinal cord, allowing for an immediate response.

The spinal cord is delicate, and twenty-six bones called vertebrae protect the spinal cord from damage. Each vertebra is sandwiched between cartilage disks, which provide cushioning, so the vertebrae do not become injured with movement or the bearing of heavy weight (Figure 2.21).

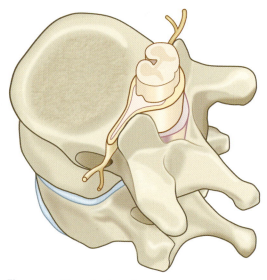

Figure 2.21 The spinal cord surrounded by the vertebrae.

Despite being encased by the vertebrae, the spinal cord is incredibly fragile and prone to injury. Damage to the spinal cord can be devastating because the injury can disrupt the flow of information traveling to and from the brain, which can cause disturbances in movement and sensation, among many other symptoms.

Automobile and motorcycle accidents are the leading cause of injury to the spinal cord, and, currently, there are no effective therapies for repairing extensive spinal cord damage (Mayo Clinic, 2021). However, researchers around the world are studying ways to replace the function of damaged nerves.

There are many experimental approaches currently in development. One strategy involves regrowing nerves using Schwann cells, which surround nerves and repair damage in the peripheral nervous system. Researchers are transplanting Schwann cells into injured regions of the spinal cord to see if the cells can repair spinal cord tissue in the central nervous system (Santamaría et al., 2018).

Another tactic involves inserting proteins that stimulate growth at the site of injury to direct the nerve cells to grow and reconnect the signaling pathway (Lu et al., 2012). Imagine the proteins leaving a trail of breadcrumbs for the axons to follow. This research is ongoing, but preliminary studies suggest it may be a viable solution.

Participating in regular exercise helps maintain spine health and prevent injury. Yoga can maintain functional stability of the spine as well as keep the back muscles engaged, strong and flexible (Omkar and Vishwas, 2009). Yoga has been shown to improve spine mobility, range of motion and flexibility in individuals regardless of age (Grabara and Szopa, 2015), and it can help to reduce back pain (Crow, Jeannot and Trewhela, 2015).

Main takeaways
- The spinal cord contains roughly one billion neurons and is involved in both involuntary and voluntary movement.
- The spinal cord is fragile, so strengthening the back and core can help to keep it safe.
- Practicing yoga can help with back stability, flexibility and pain.

EXAMPLE YOGA SEQUENCE FOR THE SPINE

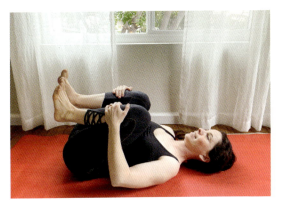

Figure 2.22 Knees to chest pose.

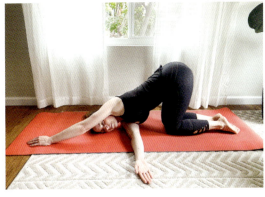

Figure 2.25 Revolved puppy dog pose.

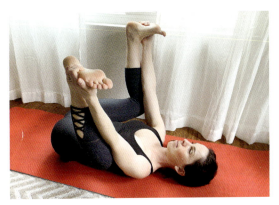

Figure 2.23 Happy baby pose.

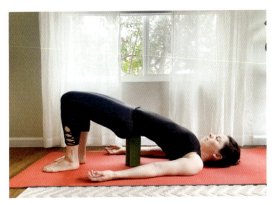

Figure 2.26 Supported bridge pose.

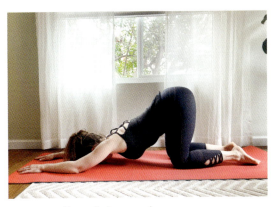

Figure 2.24 Extended puppy dog pose.

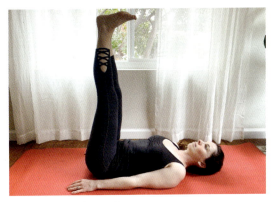

Figure 2.27 Half plough pose.

REFERENCES

Allen, N.J., & Barres, B.A., 2009. Glia: more than just brain glue. *Nature*, 457(7230), pp.675–677.

Anasuya, B., Deepak, K.K., & Jaryal, A., 2021. Yoga practitioners exhibit higher parasympathetic activity and baroreflex sensitivity and better adaptability to 40 mm Hg lower-body negative pressure. *International Journal of Yoga Therapy*, 31(1), Article_2. https://doi.org/10.17761/2021-D-20-00030.

Asare, F., Störsrud, S., & Simrén, M., 2012. Meditation over medication for irritable bowel syndrome? On exercise and alternative treatments for irritable bowel syndrome. *Current Gastroenterology Reports*, 14(4), pp.283–289.

Bardin, L., 2011. The complex role of serotonin and 5-HT receptors in chronic pain. *Behavioural Pharmacology*, 22(5 and 6), pp.390–404.

Berger, M., Gray, J.A., & Roth, B.L., 2009. The expanded biology of serotonin. *Annual Review of Medicine*, 60(1), pp.355–366.

Boonpirak, N., & Apinhasmit, W., 1994. Length and caudal level of termination of the spinal cord in Thai adults. *Cells Tissues Organs*, 149(1), pp.74–78.

Coles, J.A., 2015. Glial cells: invertebrate. *Reference Module in Biomedical Sciences*. Elsevier.

Crow, E.M., Jeannot, E., & Trewhela, A., 2015. Effectiveness of Iyengar yoga in treating spinal (back and neck) pain: a systematic review. *International Journal of Yoga*, 8(1), p.3.

Danhauer, S.C., Mihalko, S.L., Russell, G.B., Campbell, C.R., et al., 2009. Restorative yoga for women with breast cancer: findings from a randomized pilot study. *Psycho-Oncology*, 18(4), pp.360–368.

España, R.A., Schmeichel, B.E., & Berridge, C.W., 2016. Norepinephrine at the nexus of arousal, motivation and relapse. *Brain Research*, 1641, pp.207–216.

Fleming, M.A., 2nd, Ehsan, L., Moore, S.R., & Levin, D.E., 2020. The enteric nervous system and its emerging role as a therapeutic target. *Gastroenterology Research and Practice*, 2020, 8024171.

Goddard, A.W., Ball, S.G., Martinez, J., Robinson, M.J., et al., 2010. Current perspectives of the roles of the central norepinephrine system in anxiety and depression. *Depression and Anxiety*, 27(4), pp.339–350.

Goff, D.C., & Coyle, J.T., 2001. The emerging role of glutamate in the pathophysiology and treatment of schizophrenia. *American Journal of Psychiatry*, 158(9), pp.1367–1377.

Grabara, M., & Szopa, J., 2015. Effects of hatha yoga exercises on spine flexibility in women over 50 years old. *Journal of Physical Therapy Science*, 27(2), pp.361–365.

Hansen, D.V., Hanson, J.E., & Sheng, M., 2017. Microglia in Alzheimer's disease. *Journal of Cell Biology*, 217(2), pp.459–472.

Hawkins, J., & Ahmad, S., 2016. Why neurons have thousands of synapses, a theory of sequence memory in neocortex. *Frontiers in Neural Circuits*, 10, p.23.

Herculano-Houzel, S., 2012. The remarkable, yet not extraordinary, human brain as a scaled-up primate brain and its associated cost. *Proceedings of the National Academy of Sciences*, 109, pp.10661–10668.

Hodgkin, A.L., Huxley, A.F., & Katz, B., 1952. Measurement of current-voltage relations in the membrane of the giant axon of Loligo. *The Journal of Physiology*, 116(4), pp.424–448.

Jia, W., Zhen, J., Liu, A., Yuan, J., et al., 2020. Long-term vegan meditation improved human gut microbiota. *Evidence-Based Complementary and Alternative Medicine*, 7(5). doi: 10.1155/2020/9517897.

Johnson, R.L., & Wilson, C.G., 2018. A review of vagus nerve stimulation as a therapeutic intervention. *Journal of Inflammation Research*, 11, pp.203–213.

Kalueff, A.V., & Nutt, D.J., 2007. Role of GABA in anxiety and depression. *Depression and Anxiety*, 24(7), pp.495–517.

Kanaya, A.M., Araneta, M.R., Pawlowsky, S.B., Barrett-Connor, E., et al., 2014. Restorative yoga and metabolic risk factors: the Practicing Restorative Yoga vs. Stretching for the Metabolic Syndrome (PRYSMS) randomized trial. *Journal of Diabetes and its Complications*, 28(3), pp.406–412.

Kim, D.-Y., & Camilleri, M., 2000. Serotonin: a mediator of the brain-gut connection. *American Journal of Gastroenterology*, 95(10), pp.2698–2709.

Leong, H., 2019. Restorative yoga. *Physical Medicine and Rehabilitation*. Available at: https://www.med.unc.edu/phyrehab/wp-content/uploads/sites/549/2019/09/9.13.2019-Wellness.pdf

Lu, P., Wang, Y., Graham, L., McHale, K., et al., 2012. Long-distance growth and connectivity of neural stem cells after severe spinal cord injury. *Cell*, 150(6), pp.1264–1273.

Mayo Clinic, 2021. Spinal cord injury. Available at: https://www.mayoclinic.org/diseases-conditions/spinal-cord-injury/symptoms-causes/syc-20377890

McCall, C.M., 2013. How might yoga work? An overview of potential underlying mechanisms. *Journal of Yoga & Physical Therapy*, 3(1), p.130.

Nagel, S.J., Wilson, S., Johnson, M.D., Machado, A., et al., 2017. Spinal cord stimulation for spasticity: historical approaches, current status, and future directions. *Neuromodulation: Technology at the Neural Interface*, 20(4), pp.307–321.

Newman, E.A., 2003. New roles for astrocytes: regulation of synaptic transmission. *Trends in Neurosciences*, 26(10), pp.536–542.

Omkar, S.N., & Vishwas, S., 2009. Yoga techniques as a means of core stability training. *Journal of Bodywork and Movement Therapies*, 13(1), pp.98–103.

Parhi, K.K., & Unnikrishnan, N.K., 2020. Brain-inspired computing: models and architectures. *IEEE Open Journal of Circuits and Systems*, 1, pp.185–204.

Rao, M., & Gershon, M.D., 2016. The bowel and beyond: the enteric nervous system in neurological disorders. *Nature Reviews Gastroenterology & Hepatology*, 13(9), pp.517–528.

Rieder, R., Wisniewski, P.J., Alderman, B.L., & Campbell, S.C., 2017. Microbes and mental health: a review. *Brain, Behavior, and Immunity*, 66, pp.9–17.

Santamaría, A.J., Solano, J.P., Benavides, F.D., & Guest, J.D., 2018. Intraspinal delivery of Schwann cells for spinal cord injury. *Methods in Molecular Biology*, 1739, pp.467–484.

Saritas, E.U., Cunningham, C.H., Lee, J.H., Han, E.T., & Nishimura, D.G., 2008. DWI of the spinal cord with reduced FOV single-shot EPI. *Magnetic Resonance in Medicine*, 60(2), pp.468–473.

Segura-Aguilar, J., Paris, I., Muñoz, P., Ferrari, E., Zecca, L., & Zucca, F.A., 2014. Protective and toxic roles of dopamine in Parkinson's disease. *Journal of Neurochemistry*, 129(6), pp.898–915.

Si, B., & Song, E., 2018. Recent advances in the detection of neurotransmitters. *Chemosensors*, 6(1), p.1.

Starcke, K., & Brand, M., 2012. Decision making under stress: a selective review. *Neuroscience & Biobehavioral Reviews*, 36(4), pp.1228–1248.

Streeter, C.C., Gerbarg, P.L., Saper, R.B., Ciraulo, D.A., & Brown, R.P., 2012. Effects of yoga on the autonomic nervous system, gamma-aminobutyric-acid, and allostasis in epilepsy, depression, and post-traumatic stress disorder. *Medical Hypotheses*, 78(5), pp.571–579.

Tavassoli, S., 2009. Yoga in the management of irritable bowel syndrome. *International Journal of Yoga Therapy*, 19(1), pp.97–101.

Temburni, M.K., & Jacob, M.H., 2001. New functions for glia in the brain. *Proceedings of the National Academy of Sciences*, 98(7), pp.3631–3632.

Vempati, R.P., & Telles, S., 2002. Yoga-based guided relaxation reduces sympathetic activity judged from baseline levels. *Psychological Reports*, 90(2), pp.487–494.

CHAPTER 3
Anatomical Features of the Brain

> Yoga and meditation activate different regions of the brain. A significant body of research has focused on measuring the physical differences in the brains of yoga practitioners versus a control group. This chapter will explore the physical structure of the brain, its key regions as well as their basic functions.

INTRODUCTION

The human brain is a whole, connected structure. Although it largely functions as one system, anatomically it can be divided into two central hemispheres that are connected by a large bundle of nerve fibers called the corpus callosum. Each hemisphere of the brain can also be divided into four main units or lobes. The four lobes have a variety of functions and coordinate to act as one cohesive network (Figure 3.1).

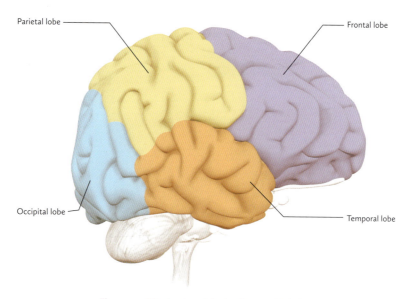

Figure 3.1 The brain with the four main lobes.

THE FRONTAL LOBE

The **frontal lobe** is located at the front of the brain (hence the name), directly behind the forehead and eyes. It is responsible for many important tasks, such as integrating information to allow for decision making. Deciding which yoga class to attend or even which leg to lift during downward-facing dog both involve the frontal lobe. The frontal lobe is also involved in motivation, attention, reward, self-control, emotional processing, personality and movement (Chayer and Freedman, 2001).

But how do neuroscientists know which regions of the brain are responsible for what? Prior to the invention of neuroimaging, the human brain was difficult to study because it is encased in a hard skull. Scientists would look at what happened to the brain when a region of it became damaged or destroyed, such as after a stroke or injury. This is exactly how scientists and doctors in the mid-1800s discovered that the frontal lobe gives rise to our personalities.

Phineas Gage

In the late 1840s, a railroad worker named Phineas Gage was blasting rock while preparing a railway in Vermont when an accident occurred. One of the blasts sent an iron rod almost 5 centimeters (2 inches) in diameter careening through the front of Gage's left cheek, directly through his frontal lobe (Figure 3.2). Gage was knocked to the ground, but he wasn't dead. To his co-workers' surprise, Gage was able to sit up and have a conversation within minutes after the accident. His survival was declared a medical miracle.

After the injury, Gage went back to everyday activities, but over time his personality began to change. He went from being a dependable, hard-working man to becoming irritable and aggressive as the years progressed. His family and friends reported that he was not the man he used to be. Gage was seen by many doctors who reasoned that the frontal lobe must be involved in personality. Despite these changes, and the hole in his brain, Gage lived another 12 years before his death in 1860.

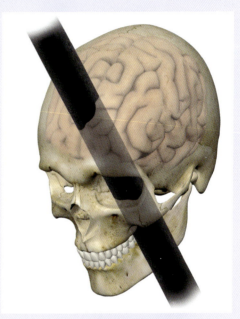

Figure 3.2 Representation of the iron rod that was shot through Gage's skull.
Source: Ratiu et al., CC BY-SA 2.1. From: https://qbi.uq.edu.au/brain/brain-anatomy/lobes-brain

Later, with the invention of neuroimaging, scientists confirmed that damage to the frontal lobe can lead to personality changes and personality disorders (Chow, 2000). After Gage's death, a doctor took possession of Gage's skull and eventually donated the skull and the iron rod to Harvard University's Warren Anatomical Museum in Boston, Massachusetts. They reside there to this day.

In the lower front portion of the frontal lobe sits the **prefrontal cortex**. It is involved in cognitive control, decision making, attention and behavior. The prefrontal cortex is one of the most studied regions of the brain, including in yoga and meditation research.

The prefrontal cortex is often associated with yoga practice. Researchers from Hospital Israelita Albert Einstein in Brazil and Harvard University found that healthy, elderly female experienced yoga practitioners have increased cortical thickness in the left prefrontal cortex when compared with a younger, activity-matched control group (Afonso et al., 2017). Cortical thickness reflects the width of the gray matter of the cortex, the outermost part of the human brain (Figure 3.3). A thicker cortex could mean that there are more healthy neurons in those areas. In contrast, a thinning cortex is a sign of neurodegeneration in certain diseases, such as Alzheimer's disease (Lerch et al., 2004).

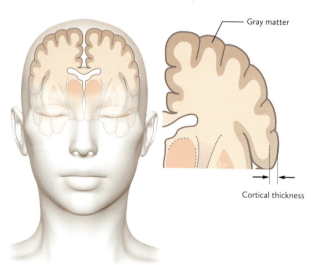

Figure 3.3 Illustration showing how scientists measure cortical thickness.

Greater cortical thickness in the prefrontal cortices of experienced yogis suggests that yoga may be able to impact the size of this important brain region. These anatomical changes could lead to functional benefits like improved cognition, decision making or impulse control, though increases in size alone don't necessarily imply improved processes.

> **Gray and white matter**
> Neuroscientists often refer to the brain as having **gray matter** and **white matter**. Gray matter contains mostly the cell bodies of neurons and their dendrites as well as glial cells and capillaries. The capillaries carry oxygenated blood to the cells, making the tissue appear pinkish in a living brain. The gray matter is found in the outer layers of the brain and in the center of the spinal cord.
>
> White matter appears white and contains mostly neuronal axons, which are the long cords that extend out from the cell body. Axons appear white due to the myelin sheath that wraps around them. The myelin helps conduct impulses of electrical signals down the axon to the terminal region of the cell to communicate with other cells. In the brain, white matter is internal to the gray matter, but in the spinal cord white matter is on the outside of the gray matter.

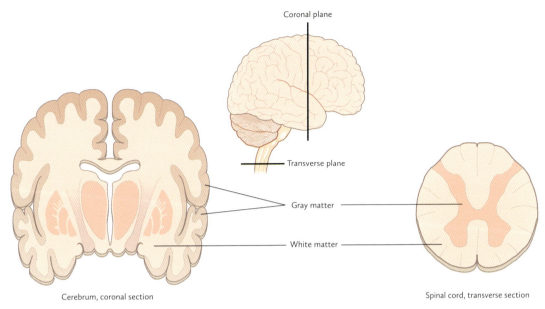

Figure 3.4 Left: Section of the brain showing gray matter on the outside and white matter on the inside. Right: Section of the spinal cord showing gray matter on the inside and white matter on the outside.

THE TEMPORAL LOBE

The **temporal lobe** is located on both sides of the brain internal to the ears. It is involved in a variety of activities including hearing, listening, language, visual processing of faces and objects as well as memory (Squire, Stark and Clark, 2004; Eichenbaum, Yonelinas and Ranganath, 2007). Although important structures are typically located bilaterally on both sides of the brain, the temporal lobe is an exception.

The left temporal lobe is home to two important structures related to language called Wernicke's area and Broca's area that are not found on the right side. Wernicke's area is responsible for the *comprehension* of speech, while Broca's area is involved in the *production* of speech. For example, when your yoga teacher provides verbal instruction, understanding the instructions requires activation of Wernicke's area. Asking a question during class uses Broca's area to conjure the words to speak. There is one exception: left-handed individuals are more likely to have their language centers located on the right side of their brain instead of the left. Neuroscientists are not entirely sure why that is the case (Knecht et al., 2000).

The temporal lobe is also involved in recognizing faces. Neuroscientist Oliver Sacks wrote a book entitled *The Man Who Mistook His Wife for a Hat* which describes a rare condition called prosopagnosia or face blindness (Sacks, 2022). People with this condition cannot recognize faces, and it is thought that this phenomenon could be due to damage of the temporal lobe. A team of scientists at Dartmouth College, Harvard University and the University of London are currently conducting a large-scale study as part of the Prosopagnosia Research Center to better understand what causes this phenomenon. They believe the condition may be due to cell death in the temporal lobe, although there is likely a genetic component involved as well.

The temporal lobe is also the brain's major

memory center. It contains the **hippocampus**, which resembles the shape of a seahorse (Figure 3.5). This region is responsible for declarative memory, which is the memory of facts and events. Some neuroscientists believe that this area can create new neurons in a process called neurogenesis (Squire, Stark and Clark, 2004; Eichenbaum, Yonelinas and Ranganath, 2007). More on neurogenesis in Chapter 10.

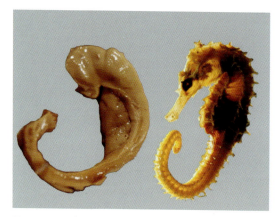

Figure 3.5 Left: Hippocampus from a human brain. Right: A seahorse resembles the shape of the hippocampus, which is where its name is derived from.
Source: Professor Laszlo Seress, CC BY-SA 3.0. From: https://theconversation.com/explainer-what-happens-in-the-hippocampus-32589

The function of the hippocampus was discovered due to a famous patient named Henry Molaison (later known as H.M.). In the early 1950s, a 26-year-old Henry underwent brain surgery that removed the majority of both of his hippocampi to curb his epileptic seizures. Although the surgery helped decrease his seizures, his memory was forever altered. He had what is called anterograde amnesia. Similar to Lucy Whitmore from *50 First Dates*, Henry could remember his childhood and most of his life, but he was unable to form new memories.

Doctors were fascinated by Henry. He underwent extensive neurological and psychological testing throughout his life after the surgery. These studies led to a better understanding of neurosurgery and allowed scientists to uncover the important role the hippocampus plays in memory formation.

Henry spent the rest of his life living in the hospital, waking up every day thinking he was a young man until he died at the age of 82 in 2008 (Annese *et al.*, 2014). Since he couldn't form new memories, he never knew how famous he had become in the field of neuroscience. After his death, researchers at the University of California, San Diego took Henry's brain and digitally reconstructed it so that neuroscientists around the world could examine his brain in stunning detail (Annese *et al.*, 2014).

How do you remember a sun salutation?

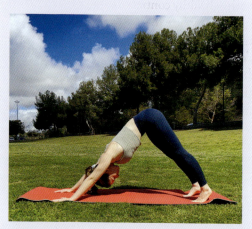

Figure 3.6 Downward-facing dog, one of the many postures in a sun salutation.

There are two main types of long-term memory: declarative (explicit memory) and nondeclarative (implicit memory). Declarative memory is how we remember facts and events, while nondeclarative memory is for habit formation and learning new skills (Reber, 2008). Henry Molaison's case taught doctors and scientists that declarative memories involve the hippocampus.

> Nondeclarative memories, like practicing a sun salutation, can operate without conscious thought once learned. These types of memories require repetition and practice for our behavior (the sun salutation) to run on autopilot. Nondeclarative memories involve movement regions of the brain, and the cerebellum plays a critical role in the execution of learned movement memories.

The hippocampus is affected by aging. As a person ages, neurons die off, inflammation increases and the hippocampus shrinks in size (Van Aalst et al., 2020). Yoga may offer protection from age-related decline. Scientists from the University of Illinois at Urbana Champaign and Wayne State University examined hippocampus density in 13 experienced yoga practitioners in comparison with 13 healthy controls (Gothe et al., 2018). They found that the experienced yogis had more gray matter density in the left hippocampus than the control group. This finding could indicate that the yogis had more neurons in this region of the brain, protecting them against age-related memory decline.

> **Why do these studies show differences in only the left side of the brain and not the right?**
> Neuroscientists do not know. A significant finding in only one side of the brain could be due to a variety of reasons including technical difficulties, errors, or differences in analysis techniques. Although some functions, like speech, are localized to the left side of the brain, most other functions are thought to occur bilaterally in the brain. However, it is possible that there are right and left side brain differences that have yet to be discovered.

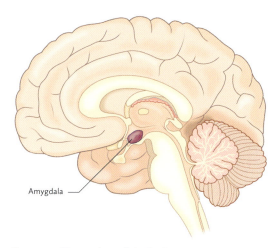

Figure 3.7 Illustration of the brain showing the amygdala.

The hippocampus is located next to the **amygdala** (Figure 3.7). Each amygdala is roughly the shape and size of an almond. Despite being so small, these structures play a major role processing fear, anxiety and anger. The amygdala also attaches emotions to our memories and, thus, is a central relay station for emotional memory (Van Aalst et al., 2020).

Researchers at the Erasmus Medical Center in the Netherlands examined the effect of yoga and meditation on volume of the amygdala and hippocampus in a large study of 3,742 participants (Gotink et al., 2018). They found that a decrease in gray matter volume in the left hippocampus and the right amygdala was associated with both practices. Less gray matter volume in these regions could signify that the practitioner uses yoga and meditation to control their emotional state to regulate the anxiety and fear response. If the neurons related to anxiety and fear were not being used as often, the brain could have reorganized these circuits, decreasing the volume of these regions. This process may help the brain become more efficient. The scientists did not make a distinction between the effect of yoga vs. meditation on the brain, so it is unclear if the results were due to yoga, meditation or both practices combined.

Is it better to have more or less gray matter volume?

Both options seem to have plausible benefits. One of the main difficulties in determining the answer is that brain volume is based on imaging studies and not on dissection studies. Thus, it is unclear what is causing the size differences. Researchers are starting to approach this question by dissecting the brains of animal models, such as mice and rats, to see how brain volume is related to brain structure.

Do more intelligent people have bigger brains?

It is commonly believed that a larger brain must equate to more intelligence, but consider the African elephant. It has a brain that is approximately three times the size of a human brain. An elephant's brain contains nearly 257 billion neurons in comparison with a human's meager 86 billion neurons (Herculano-Houzel *et al.*, 2014).

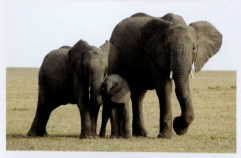

Figure 3.8 African elephants in Masai Mara National Reserve, Kenya.
Source: David Heiling on Unsplash.

Careful examination of Albert Einstein's brain has revealed that his brain was actually smaller than the typical human brain (Costandi, 2012). Dissection studies have shown that his brain was denser, meaning that Einstein had more neurons densely packed together in regions across his brain.

A denser brain could signify that Einstein had more connectivity between brain regions, enabling faster processing than the average brain. Einstein also had more nonneuronal support cells, called glia, than the average human brain (Costandi, 2012). Neuroscientists are still trying to figure out how glia could be related to intelligence.

Left-brained or right-brained dominant?

There is little truth to the statement "right-brained people are creative or artistic, while left-brained people are more analytical or calculating." While some brain functions, such as language, are localized to one side of the brain, most brain functions occur bilaterally. Information is shared through a bridge of 300 million axons called the corpus callosum (Phillips *et al.*, 2015). The **corpus callosum** is a highway for information traveling to and from the right and left hemispheres of the brain.

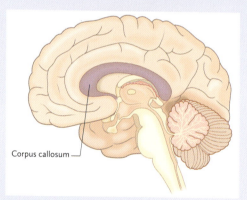

Figure 3.9 Illustration of the brain showing the corpus callosum.

Sometimes this bridge must be severed. In conditions like severe epilepsy, neurologists will cut the corpus callosum so that the two hemispheres of the brain can no longer communicate with one another. This surgery can decrease seizures, but it can also lead to a host of behavioral and cognitive changes, such as alterations in vision, speech and memory. It is considered a last resort surgery, reserved for patients without an alternative treatment option.

So, why are some people more creative or analytical? Neuroscientists don't know, but it could have to do with how groups of neurons communicate with one another.

THE PARIETAL LOBE

The **parietal lobe** is located near the back and top of the brain, and it specializes in processing sensory information such as taste, touch, temperature, pain and pressure (Garcia-Larrea and Mauguière, 2018). It also integrates this sensory information with the visual system, which is important for knowing where the body is in space, called proprioception (Karnath, 1997; Olson and Berryhill, 2009). Also known as the sixth sense, proprioception is critical for almost every type of movement. One study showed that the volume of the parietal lobe was related to the weekly number of hours spent practicing yoga. Yogis that practiced yoga more often had larger parietal lobes than those who practiced less frequently (Villemure *et al.*, 2015).

THE OCCIPITAL LOBE

The smallest lobe, the **occipital lobe**, is located all the way in the back of the brain, and it is home to the main visual processing center, the primary visual cortex. The occipital lobe is located far from our eyes, so the brain has evolved to have millions of axons (white matter) that extend from the eyes to the occipital lobe. The occipital lobe integrates information from the eyes to form one cohesive image with information about light, texture, color, size, shape and distance.

Underneath the occipital lobe lie two more important structures called the cerebellum and the brainstem (Figure 3.10). The **cerebellum**, which means "little brain" in Latin, is involved in coordinating movements, muscle memory (like a sun salutation), movement correction (quick movements to avoid tripping) as well as a host of other functions neuroscientists are just starting to decipher. Although it is physically smaller than the cerebral cortex, it contains roughly five times as many neurons that are densely packed into this wrinkly space (Von Bartheld, Bahney and Herculano-Houzel, 2016).

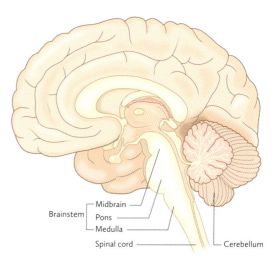

Figure 3.10 Illustration of the brain showing the brainstem, cerebellum and spinal cord.
Adapted from: https://qbi.uq.edu.au/brain/brain-anatomy/hindbrain

The **brainstem** regulates many important functions, such as breathing, heart rate, blood pressure, consciousness and sleep–wake cycles. The brainstem consists of three main sections called the midbrain, pons and medulla oblongata, which is often shortened to "medulla." Long-term meditation has been shown to increase the density of the brainstem, specifically in regions associated with heart and lung control (Vestergaard-Poulsen *et al.*, 2009). These brain structure changes could account for the increased parasympathetic nervous system activity that is often correlated with meditation.

The brainstem is also home to most of the brain's cranial nerves. Cranial nerves each have a specific role in transmitting movement and/or sensory information around the head and neck (Figure 3.11).

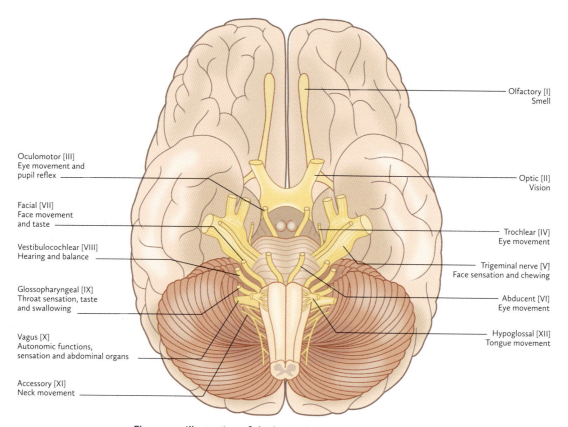

Figure 3.11 Illustration of the brain showing the cranial nerves.

The **midbrain** is the top portion of the brainstem and is involved with the control of movement, sleep, temperature regulation, vision and hearing. It contains the main dopamine production center called the substantia nigra.

The **pons** is located between the midbrain and the medulla. This bulbous structure gets its name from the Latin word for "bridge" as it serves as a coordination center for signals coming to and from both sides of the brain as well as the spinal cord. The pons contains groups of neurons that are involved in sleep, respiration, equilibrium and many more functions.

The **medulla** is the lowest portion of the brainstem, and this is where the brain transitions into the spinal cord. Although the medulla is short, measuring roughly 3 centimeters (1 inch) long, it is a critical structure for our survival. It contains control centers for vital functions, such as breathing, heart rate and blood pressure. This region is also involved in reflexes like swallowing and even sneezing (Seijo-Martinez *et al.*, 2006; Hashimoto *et al.*, 2018).

ADDITIONAL BRAIN REGIONS RELEVANT TO YOGA AND MEDITATION

The cingulate cortex curls around the inside of the brain like a rainbow (Figure 3.12). It is divided into two main sections, the anterior cingulate cortex (the front portion) and the posterior cingulate cortex (the back portion).

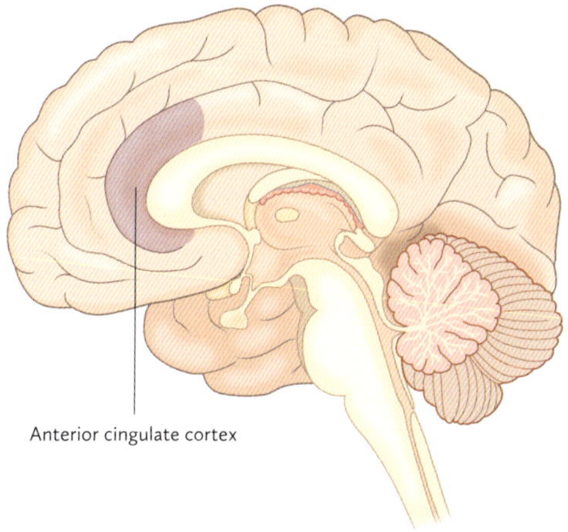

(Figure 3.13). Scientists believe it is responsible for self-awareness and self-reflection, as it senses the interior state of the body (Modinos, Ormel and Aleman, 2009).

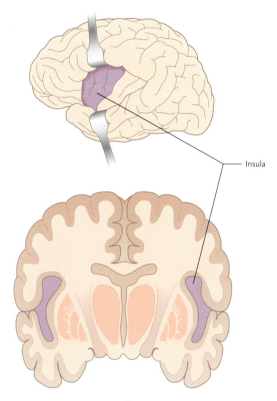

Figure 3.12 Illustration of the brain showing the anterior cingulate cortex.

The **anterior cingulate cortex** (ACC) is especially relevant for yoga practitioners because it is connected to the emotional system of the brain (the limbic system) as well as the frontal lobe that is responsible for making decisions. The ACC helps to integrate thoughts and feelings for emotional learning as well as monitor focus during activities like meditation (Devinsky, Morrell and Vogt, 1995).

The ACC is commonly associated with the effects of meditation. Meditation can increase the efficiency of this region, improve blood flow and induce axonal changes (Tang et al., 2010, 2015; Xue, Tang and Posner, 2011). Some researchers hypothesize that changes in these regions of the brain could lead to improved emotional and attentional regulation.

The **insula** or insular cortex has recently taken the spotlight in meditation research

Figure 3.13 Illustration of the brain showing the insula or insular cortex.

Multiple studies have found that yoga practitioners have larger insular volumes (gray matter) than non-yoga practitioners. The size of the insula is also related to years of yoga experience; people who have been practicing yoga for longer periods of time have more gray matter in this region than less experienced yoga practitioners (Villemure et al., 2013).

Another way to explore the brain is by looking at neurons' axons called the white matter. Examining white matter is useful for understanding how different areas of the brain are connected. Researchers from the National Institutes of Health were interested in how the white matter differed in the insulas of experienced yoga practitioners in comparison with healthy controls (Villemure *et al.*, 2013). Experienced practitioners showed more connectivity between the front (anterior) and back (posterior) regions of the insula than the control subjects. Yoga requires mind and body awareness, so this practice could be altering the insula to promote efficient communication, making awareness and self-reflection more accessible.

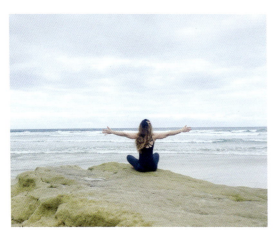

Figure 3.14 Loving-kindness meditation trains the brain to cultivate compassion, forgiveness and self-acceptance.

The insula is also involved with feeling empathy, and it is believed to be activated during loving-kindness meditation (LKM) (Singer, Critchley and Preuschoff, 2009). LKM is a popular meditation technique used to boost well-being and reduce stress (Figure 3.14). It trains the brain to cultivate compassion, forgiveness and self-acceptance. During LKM, the meditator focuses on bringing loving, kind energy to another person or themselves. Although this technique can be difficult to master, it can promote better emotional regulation and stress management (Grossman and Van Dam, 2011).

Loving-kindness meditation

Bring yourself to a comfortable position.
Let's start by cultivating loving kindness for a friend or family member.
Someone you love.
Think about your desire for
them to be happy.
A natural opening of the heart outward.
Check in with your body and how
you're feeling in this moment.
Be here and now. Let the
feelings rest in place.
Now, start to focus on the
loved person again.
Try to visualize their appearance.
Take in their smells.
Remember the way they move their body.
Sense them, see them.
Now, notice how you're feeling inside.
Start to cultivate that warmth.
Are you smiling?
Happiness is a natural feeling.
Bring that loved one back
to your attention.
Wish them well and send them love.
May you be happy, healthy and peaceful.
Feel the loving kindness
extend from yourself.
Feel your inner strength and fire.
Imagine extending joy and happiness to your loved person.
May we all experience joy and happiness.

Main takeaways
- Although the brain relies on many different regions working together to function, we've learned that some areas are responsible for the bulk of certain functions (Figure 3.15).
- Scientific studies have linked the practice of yoga and meditation to changes in almost every region of the brain.

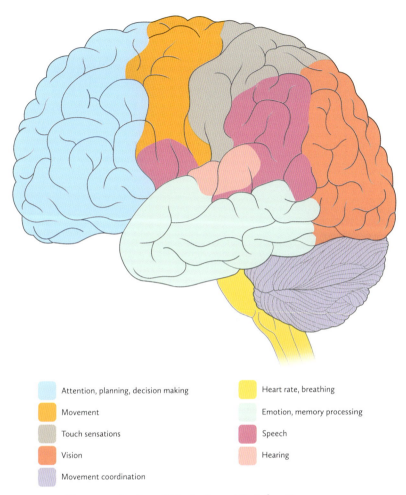

Figure 3.15 Regions of the brain and their functions.

REFERENCES

Afonso, R.F., Balardin, J.B., Lazar, S., Sato, J., et al., 2017. Greater cortical thickness in elderly female yoga practitioners: a cross-sectional study. *Frontiers in Aging Neuroscience*, 9, p.201.

Annese, J., Schenker-Ahmed, N.M., Bartsch, H., Maechler, P., et al., 2014. Postmortem examination of patient H.M.'s brain based on histological sectioning and digital 3D reconstruction. *Nature Communications*, 5(1), p.3122.

Chayer, C., & Freedman, M., 2001. Frontal lobe functions. *Current Neurology and Neuroscience Reports*, 1(6), pp.547–552.

Chow, T.W., 2000. Personality in frontal lobe disorders. *Current Psychiatry Reports*, 2(5), pp.446–451.

Costandi, M., 2012. Snapshots explore Einstein's unusual brain. *Nature*. https://doi.org/10.1038/nature.2012.11836.

Devinsky, O., Morrell, M.J., & Vogt, B.A., 1995. Contributions of anterior cingulate cortex to behaviour. *Brain*, 118(1), pp.279–306.

Eichenbaum, H., Yonelinas, A.P., & Ranganath, C., 2007. The medial temporal lobe and recognition memory. *Annual Review of Neuroscience*, 30(1), pp.123–152.

Garcia-Larrea, L., & Mauguière, F., 2018. Pain syndromes and the parietal lobe. *Handbook of Clinical Neurology*, 151, pp.207–223.

Gothe, N.P., Hayes, J.M., Temali, C., & Damoiseaux, J.S., 2018. Differences in brain structure and function among yoga practitioners and controls. *Frontiers in Integrative Neuroscience*, 12, p.26.

Gotink, R.A., Vernooij, M.W., Ikram, M.A., Niessen, W.J., et al., 2018. Meditation and yoga practice are associated with smaller right amygdala volume: The Rotterdam Study. *Brain Imaging and Behavior*, 12(6), pp.1631–1639.

Grossman, P., & Van Dam, N.T., 2011. Mindfulness, by any other name...: Trials and tribulations of Sati in western psychology and science. *Contemporary Buddhism*, 12(1), pp.219–239.

Hashimoto, K., Sugiyama, Y., Fuse, S., Umezaki, T., et al., 2018. Activity of swallowing-related neurons in the medulla in the perfused brainstem preparation in rats. *The Laryngoscope*, 129(2), e72–e79.

Herculano-Houzel, S., Avelino-de-Souza, K., Neves, K., Porfírio, J., et al., 2014. The elephant brain in numbers. *Frontiers in Neuroanatomy*, 8, p.46.

Karnath, H.O., 1997. Spatial orientation and the representation of space with parietal lobe lesions. *Philosophical Transactions of the Royal Society of London. Series B: Biological Sciences*, 352(1360), pp.1411–1419.

Knecht, S., Dräger, B., Deppe, M., Bobe, L., et al., 2000. Handedness and hemispheric language dominance in healthy humans. *Brain*, 123(12), pp.2512–2518.

Lerch, J.P., Pruessner, J.C., Zijdenbos, A., Hampel, H., Teipel, S.J., & Evans, A.C., 2004. Focal decline of cortical thickness in Alzheimer's disease identified by computational neuroanatomy. *Cerebral Cortex*, 15(7), pp.995–1001.

Modinos, G., Ormel, J., & Aleman, A., 2009. Activation of anterior insula during self-reflection. *PLoS ONE*, 4(2), e4618.

Olson, I.R., & Berryhill, M., 2009. Some surprising findings on the involvement of the parietal lobe in human memory. *Neurobiology of Learning and Memory*, 91(2), pp.155–165.

Phillips, K.A., Stimpson, C.D., Smaers, J.B., Raghanti, M.A., et al., 2015. The corpus callosum in primates: processing speed of axons and the evolution of hemispheric asymmetry. *Proceedings of the Royal Society B: Biological Sciences*, 282(1818), p.20151535.

Reber, P.J., 2008. Cognitive neuroscience of declarative and nondeclarative memory. *Advances in Psychology*, 139, pp.113–123.

Sacks, O., 2022. *The Man Who Mistook His Wife for a Hat*. London: Picador.

Seijo-Martinez, M., Varela-Freijanes, A., Grandes, J., & Vázquez, F., 2006. Sneeze related area in the medulla: localisation of the human sneezing centre? *Journal of Neurology, Neurosurgery & Psychiatry*, 77(4), pp.559–561.

Singer, T., Critchley, H.D., & Preuschoff, K., 2009. A common role of insula in feelings, empathy and uncertainty. *Trends in Cognitive Sciences*, 13(8), pp.334–340.

Squire, L.R., Stark, C.E.L., & Clark, R.E., 2004. The medial temporal lobe. *Annual Review of Neuroscience*, 27(1), pp.279–306.

Tang, Y.-Y., Lu, Q., Geng, X., Stein, E.A., Yang, Y., & Posner, M.I., 2010. Short-term meditation induces white matter changes in the anterior cingulate. *Proceedings of the National Academy of Sciences*, 107(35), pp.15649–15652.

Tang, Y.-Y., Lu, Q., Feng, H., Tang, R., & Posner, M.I., 2015. Short-term meditation increases blood flow in anterior cingulate cortex and insula. *Frontiers in Psychology*, 6, p.212.

Van Aalst, J., Ceccarini, J., Demyttenaere, K., Sunaert, S., & Van Laere, K., 2020. What has neuroimaging taught us on the neurobiology of yoga? A review. *Frontiers in Integrative Neuroscience*, 14, p.34.

Vestergaard-Poulsen, P., van Beek, M., Skewes, J., Bjarkam, C.R., et al., 2009. Long-term meditation is associated with increased gray matter density in the brain stem. *NeuroReport*, 20(2), pp.170–174.

Villemure, C., Ceko, M., Cotton, V.A., & Bushnell, M.C., 2013. Insular cortex mediates increased pain tolerance in yoga practitioners. *Cerebral Cortex*, 24(10), pp.2732–2740.

Villemure, C., Ceko, M., Cotton, V.A., & Bushnell, M.C., 2015. Neuroprotective effects of yoga practice: age-, experience-, and frequency-dependent plasticity. *Frontiers in Human Neuroscience*, 9, p.281.

Von Bartheld, C.S., Bahney, J., & Herculano-Houzel, S., 2016. The search for true numbers of neurons and glial cells in the human brain: a review of 150 years of cell counting. *Journal of Comparative Neurology*, 524(18), pp.3865–3895.

Xue, S., Tang, Y.-Y., & Posner, M.I., 2011. Short-term meditation increases network efficiency of the anterior cingulate cortex. *NeuroReport*, 22(12), pp.570–574.

CHAPTER 4

The Sensory Experience of Yoga and Meditation

The senses are a fundamental part of every yoga and meditation experience. They are the portals by which the body perceives the external environment. Incorporating the senses into practice can intensify the experience and lead to vivid memories. This chapter provides a short overview of each of the senses and how they serve as sensors of the brain. This knowledge can deepen the impact of your own practice (Figure 4.1).

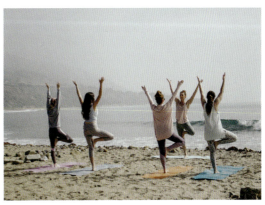

Figure 4.1 Group yoga practice on the beach.
Source: Kaylee Garrett on Unsplash.

SIGHT

When walking into a yoga studio and looking around to find a spot, thousands of signals are being sent from the neurons in the eyes to the visual center of the brain – the visual cortex. These neurons continue to send information while watching the instructor at the front of the room and glancing at the body to make sure alignment is correct. We often rely on the eyes during yoga practice, but how does vision work?

The eyes are the first part of the body to process light. When light enters the eye, it passes through the cornea, a clear and protective outer layer, which helps initially focus the light. Light then moves through the lens, which provides a more fine-tuned focusing to project the light onto the retina in the back of the eye. The iris and the pupil control how much light is let into the back of the eye (Figure 4.2).

The retina is covered in roughly 125–150 million neurons called **photoreceptors** that gather information about the incoming light and turn the information into electrical signals (Alexiades and Khanal, 2007). The photoreceptors then relay these signals to other neurons in the retina.

The two main types of photoreceptors are called rods and cones. Rods are sensitive to light and help us see at night or in dimly lit areas, whereas cones are responsible for color vision and details. There are three types of cones that detect red, green and blue colors, just like the colors of the screen pixels in a television or computer monitor. Cones work together to convey information about every detectable color.

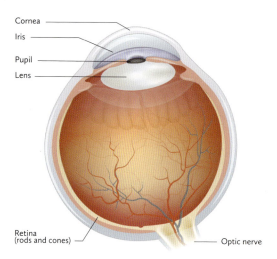

Figure 4.2 The anatomy of the eye.

The neurons in the retina then send signals to the optic nerve which transports the information along the optic tract to the visual cortex of the occipital lobe. The brain doesn't just code for shapes, movement and colors; it is able to take this visual information and use it to build memories of our visual experiences. The visual cortex sends signals to the parietal lobe for processing "where" things are in space. It also sends signals to the temporal lobe for processing "what" information, such as objects and faces. The processing in the temporal lobe is strongly connected with memory centers, including the hippocampus.

Blindness and visual impairment
Blindness and visual impairment can be caused by numerous factors, including genetics, injury and age-related changes like cataracts and glaucoma. Visual impairment can be mild, moderate or severe, with blindness being near-to-none or no vision.

Vision is not necessary to practice yoga. For some yogis, not relying on the eyes can make turning the attention inward more accessible.

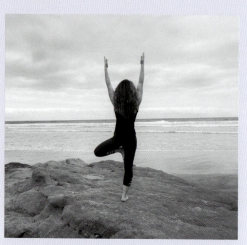

Figure 4.3 Tree pose.

When teaching yoga to blind, low-vision or visually impaired individuals, there are a few things to keep in mind. For example, a yoga study of blind and low-vision adolescents showed that students preferred physical guidance of asanas over other instructional strategies (Mohanty et al., 2016).

Tips for teaching those with blindness or vision impairment

- Use descriptive verbal cues during class.
- If the student gives permission, offer physical guidance.
- Check in with your students by asking "how does it feel?"
- Use props or scents to heighten the other senses.

THE THIRD EYE

Many practitioners and spiritual healers believe that, in addition to the physical eyes, there is also a symbolic third eye that rests in the middle of the forehead. Although this perspective does not easily align with Western medicine, according to yogic tradition the physical eyes look outward at the world, while the third eye is turned inward. The idea of a third eye exists across many different cultures and religions, such as the wisdom eye which is seen in many deities in Buddhism and the god Shiva in Hinduism. The third eye represents consciousness, spiritual knowledge and wisdom.

The concept of the third eye is also a vital part of the chakras, which are seven vortexes of energy distributed throughout the body (Figure 4.4). In yogic tradition, the third eye chakra, also called ajna chakra, can help with visualization, spiritual communication and intuition. Some believe it can establish a connection between the internal and external worlds. When the third eye chakra is open and flowing, it can provide clarity and insight. An imbalance in this chakra is thought to cause issues with the eyes or vision, as well as insomnia and headaches (Jain, 2020).

According to yogic tradition, the pineal gland is considered the biological component of the third eye. The pineal gland is a small gland deep within the brain that processes information about light and dark. Thus, it acts like a "third eye" to sense the world. The pineal gland weighs less than 0.2 grams, and it secretes serotonin, melatonin and N,N-dimethyltryptamine, which affect the body in numerous ways (Nichols, 2017; Gheban, Rosca and Crisan, 2019). The small gland has specialized cells that help regulate the 24-hour sleep–wake cycle (called the circadian rhythm) by secreting the hormone melatonin (Malpaux et al., 2001). Melatonin is secreted during periods of darkness and suppressed by light.

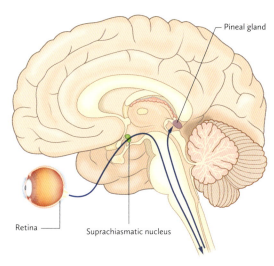

Figure 4.5 The retina, suprachiasmatic nucleus of the hypothalamus and the pineal gland.

When light hits the retina of the eye, information about vision is sent to a group of neurons in the hypothalamus called the suprachiasmatic nucleus, which is the body's internal clock (Moore, Speh and Leak, 2002). From the suprachiasmatic nucleus, information is sent to a group of neurons called the superior cervical ganglion in the neck before the information is

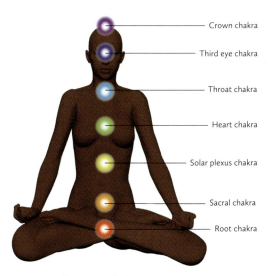

Figure 4.4 The seven chakras.

transmitted to the pineal gland (Moore, 1995) (Figure 4.5).

The pineal gland also secrets *N,N*-dimethyltryptamine (DMT), an extremely powerful hallucinogen. Some neuroscientists believe DMT is secreted during the experience of being born, giving birth and just before death (Gheban, Rosca and Crisan, 2019), while other scientists insist that the amount of DMT secreted by the pineal gland is not enough to have any psychoactive effects (Nichols, 2017). Yet, the release of DMT in the brain is implicated in near-death experiences, where people report experiencing supernatural phenomena. DMT could provide another avenue linking the physiological with the spiritual, but this has not been scientifically proven.

Main takeaways
- Photoreceptors in the eyes relay signals to the occipital lobe providing visual information.
- Descriptive verbal cues and physical guidance are helpful instructional strategies when leading classes for the visually impaired.
- The third eye chakra is linked to the pineal gland, which regulates the circadian rhythm.

Postures that place a focus on the third eye are thought to awaken the third eye chakra. This includes postures that physically touch the middle of the forehead as well as those that bring the forehead to the floor to provide gentle pressure to this region. Below is an example class of some postures that may help to ignite the anja chakra to bring forth clarity, insight and wisdom.

EXAMPLE YOGA SEQUENCE TO STIMULATE THE THIRD EYE CHAKRA

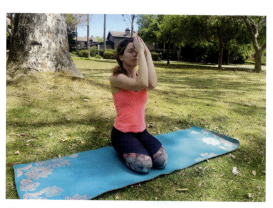

Figure 4.6 Kneeling with thumbs pressed into the third eye.

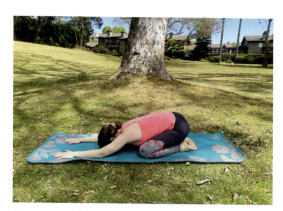

Figure 4.7 Child's pose.

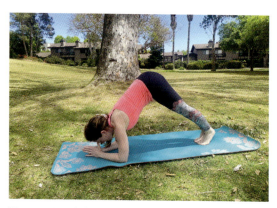

Figure 4.8 Dolphin pose variation.

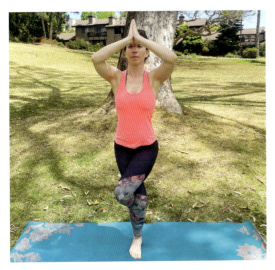

Figure 4.9 Eagle pose variation.

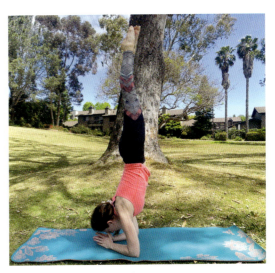

Figure 4.10 Forearm stand variation.

HEARING

Listening to the instructions of a yoga teacher or hearing "Om" during a group meditation are vital parts of many contemplative practices. In order to hear sound, the brain processes sound waves, which are transmitted and amplified through a series of membranes, liquid and bones.

The first obstacle a sound wave encounters is the eardrum (also called the tympanic membrane). When the sound waves hit the eardrum, the membrane begins to vibrate. This process transforms sound waves into vibrations. The inner ear contains three small bones called the malleus (meaning mallet), incus (meaning anvil) and stapes (meaning stirrup) that help detect these vibrations. Collectively, the three bones are known as the auditory ossicles (Figure 4.11).

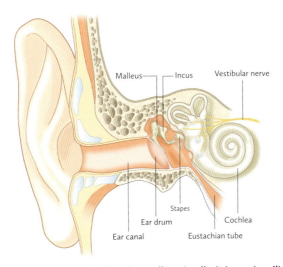

Figure 4.11 The auditory ossicles including the malleus (mallet), incus (anvil) and stapes (stirrup).

Hearing loss, deafness and hearing devices

Hearing loss and deafness can occur due to many reasons, including genetic factors, infections of the inner ear or trauma to the head. Hearing loss can be mild, moderate, severe or profound, whereas deafness is usually defined as little-to-no hearing.

You have likely worked with a student who wore a hearing aid or cochlear implant. Hearing aids help those with hearing loss by amplifying sounds to make them louder. Cochlear implants are worn by those who have significant hearing loss. The implant works by placing a processor behind the ear and a receiver in the cochlea of the inner ear. When the processor captures a sound signal, it sends it to the receiver, which stimulates the auditory nerve to send a signal to the brain.

Yoga and meditation can reduce symptoms of tinnitus, a ringing in the ear that is associated with hearing loss, and improve the daily life of deaf and hard-of-hearing individuals (Curtis and Leppla, 2018; Gunjawate and Ravi, 2021).

Tips for teaching those with hearing loss or deafness

- Help the student find a central spot in the room, so they can visually observe others' movements.
- Provide visual cues, in addition to verbal cues, during class.
- Face the student when you speak, so they can lip-read.
- Keep the lights on during class, so that interpreting visual cues and lip-reading is possible.

The vibrations first hit the malleus, which is connected to both the eardrum and the incus. The malleus moves back and forth due to the vibrations of the eardrum. This action moves the incus, which presses on the stapes. The stapes pushes against the cochlea, creating waves of fluid inside the cochlea.

Tiny, specialized cells called hair cells then sense the motion of the fluid and release neurotransmitters. The neurotransmitters signal to the neurons to fire, and information about the sound is passed on to the auditory cortex, located in the temporal lobe of the brain. After this initial processing, the information is then sent to other regions of the brain, such as the frontal cortex, to further interpret the sound signals.

Music and the brain

Yoga teachers often use music to set the mood of a class, and listening to music affects the brain in complex ways. Music triggers the brain's reward pathway, which releases the neurotransmitter dopamine. Dopamine can bring about the sense of euphoria, which is why listening to music can be pleasurable.

Music also activates memory centers in the brain. Scientists have found that listening to a favorite song alters the communication between auditory brain areas and the hippocampus, a region that connects memories with emotions (Wilkins *et al.*, 2014). This brain connection makes it easy to remember the lyrics to a favorite song.

Music therapy and sound baths

Sound has been used for thousands of years across cultures as a way of healing. Music therapy is thought to be one of the oldest forms of healing known to us (Heather, 2007). It can provide benefits to people experiencing a variety of conditions, including depression (Erkkilä *et al.*, 2011), anxiety (Gómez Gallego and Gómez García, 2017), neurological disorders, such as Parkinson's disease (Devlin, Alshaikh and Pantelyat, 2019), autism (Geretsegger *et al.*, 2014) and those recovering from traumatic brain injuries (Siponkoski *et al.*, 2020).

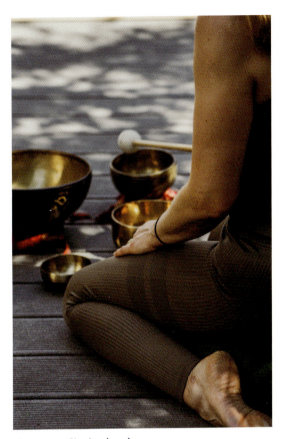

Figure 4.12 Singing bowls.
Source: Sven Mieke on Unsplash.

Despite the long history of use and many studies showing its merits, the evidence behind why sound benefits the body remains scarce. Some researchers have argued that the voice, drumming, tuning forks, singing bowls or other instruments align the body's frequencies (Figure 4.12). Researchers at the University of California, Santa Barbara developed a "resonance theory of consciousness" that describes how synchronized vibrations bring about consciousness through neurons firing at specific frequencies (Hunt, 2018). When two objects are brought into close proximity to one another, they synchronize to the same frequency in a process called "spontaneous self-organization." Music may help to shift these vibrations, bringing about a harmonious, calming effect (Heather, 2007).

Sound may be able to synchronize the firing of neurons by providing a stable frequency (Abhang, Gawali and Mehrotra, 2016; Martinez, 2021). A practitioner may be able to alter the frequency and rhythm of the sound to change the brain's waves from fluctuating at a beta state (awake) to alpha (relaxed) or theta (meditative) states (Martinez, 2021). However, more research needs to be conducted to confirm these findings.

Another type of sound healing is guided meditation, in which the voice of a practitioner or teacher acts as the sound. Guided meditation elicits the relaxation response, shifting the body into a place of calm. Many studies have shown that guided meditation promotes mental, emotional and physical well-being (Melville *et al.*, 2012).

Chanting

Chanting has been used for thousands of years around the globe to promote relaxation, a sense of community and spirituality. Chanting is considered a focused attention meditative technique, as the practitioner directs their attention towards the sound (Simpson, Perry and Thompson, 2021). The sound is also called a mantra, and it can be repeated verbally or silently.

Although there have been relatively few studies on the effects of chanting on the brain, the literature does suggest that chanting can help to decrease stress as well as improve symptoms of anxiety (Amin *et al.*, 2016; Rankhambe and Pande, 2021), depression (Kenny, Bernier and DeMartini, 2005; Amin *et al.*, 2016) and post-traumatic stress disorder (Bormann *et al.*, 2018). Chanting may be able to impact the parasympathetic nervous system by slowing the breath and activating the vagus nerve. One small study conducted by researchers from the Alzheimer's Research and Prevention Foundation in Arizona found blood flow changes in the brain during chanting (Khalsa *et al.*, 2009). Although it was a preliminary study with only 11 participants, the researchers believe that chanting increased blood flow in the same regions of the brain associated with the deterioration seen in

Alzheimer's disease. Thus, chanting could provide a neuroprotective effect in these areas of the brain.

Researchers from Macquarie University in Sydney, Australia are actively examining the effects of chanting on the body and mind. They have found that chanting "Om" for 10 minutes improves attention, mood and feelings of social cohesion (Perry, Polito and Thompson, 2016). When the scientists compared silent chanting with vocal chanting, they found that both practices led to increases in feelings of altruism.

Most recently the group of scientists explored the idea of using vocal chanting as a virtual psychosocial intervention (Simpson, Perry and Thompson, 2021). Although most chanting practices take place in social contexts, due to the coronavirus pandemic many chanting practices were moved online to adhere to social distancing guidelines. The scientists wanted to know if online chanting practices brought about the same benefits as an in-person practice. They assessed the effects of a 10-minute online chanting practice on stress, mood and connectedness.

Over 100 people participated in the study. Compared with an online task control group, the online chanting group reported a significant reduction in stress and an improvement in mood. The online chanters also felt a greater sense of connectedness to other members of the group than the control group reported. The study suggests that online chanting may be an accessible option for boosting mental health.

> **Main takeaways**
> - To hear sound, the brain processes sound waves, which are transmitted and amplified through a series of membranes, liquid and bones.
> - When teaching someone with hearing loss, provide visual and verbal cues during class. Remember to face the person during class, so that they can lip-read.
> - Sound therapy and guided meditation promote mental, emotional and physical well-being.
> - Chanting can improve stress, anxiety, attention, mood and connectedness.

SMELL

Smell is one of the most important ways humans interact with the world, yet this sense is often underappreciated. Without the sense of smell, incense and essential oils (Figure 4.13) become undetectable, and food like chocolate becomes tasteless.

How the brain smells

The ability to smell relies on a process of sensing chemicals called **chemosensation**. Inside the back of the nose is a specialized strip of tissue called the olfactory epithelium that houses millions of sensory neurons called olfactory receptor cells (Figure 4.14). These cells have tiny tips called cilia full of receptors that stick out into the nasal cavity to detect smells that enter through the nose.

> **Do humans have a bad sense of smell?**
> There is a common misconception that humans have a limited sense of smell when compared with animals, such as dogs (Yong, 2017). This idea arose from 19th-century neuroscientist Paul Broca, the same person who discovered Broca's area. He thought the sense of smell was animalistic (Shulman, 2018). Broca was convinced that humans could only detect 10,000 different types of smells; however, neuroscientists today

believe that humans are able to detect closer to one trillion different types of smells (Bushdid *et al.*, 2014).

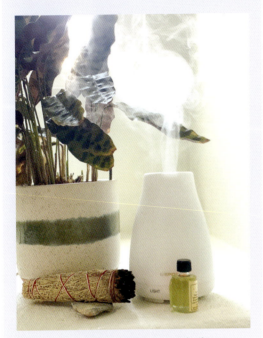

Figure 4.13 A diffuser with essential oil.

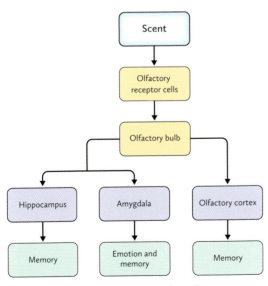

Figure 4.14 The neural pathway of smell.

When the olfactory receptor cells sense a chemical, a signal is sent to the olfactory bulb, a structure that relays the signal to other areas of the brain for processing. Most smell processing occurs in the olfactory cortex, which is located in the temporal lobe of the brain.

A portion of the olfactory cortex is called the piriform cortex, and it helps identify categories of smells, like fruity or minty (Bao *et al.*, 2016). The signals are also sent to the bottom portion of the prefrontal cortex, the orbitofrontal cortex, where the smell information is integrated with taste information (Rolls, 2008). Smell is thought to be the only sense that is not processed by the thalamus, the main brain processing center, although research is still ongoing (Courtiol and Wilson, 2015).

Smells and memory

Smell information is also sent to the brain's learning and memory centers, the hippocampus and the amygdala. The hippocampus processes long-term memories, while the amygdala processes emotional memories. These regions of the brain work to integrate information about smell with memories, such as remembering a significant other when catching a whiff of their cologne or feeling relaxed when inhaling lavender essential oil at the end of a yoga class.

Essential oils

Smells can also be used to promote health and well-being. The practice of using essential oils for therapeutic benefit, called aromatherapy, is used in healthcare settings and yoga studios. In the clinic, aromatherapy can reduce levels of anxiety and depression, as well as improve symptoms of chronic pain and increase sleep (Ali *et al.*, 2015). These strong scents can also trigger emotional responses, such as relaxation, when used in a constructive manner.

In the studio, essential oils can be used in a variety of capacities to benefit the practitioner. A few drops of an essential oil can be added to a diffuser or mixed with water and sprayed to bring soothing scents into the room. Diluted essential oils can also be rubbed directly onto the wrists, feet or forehead for an additional scent experience (Figure 4.15).

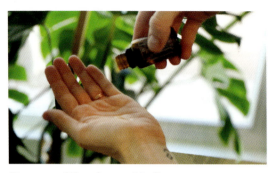

Figure 4.15 Diluted essential oil dropped into the hand.

Some popular essentials oils include:

- **Lavender oil** can help to relieve stress and digestive distress, reduce anxiety and inflammation, and promote sleep. It also has antibacterial and antifungal properties (Ali *et al.*, 2015).
- **Tea tree oil** has natural antiseptic properties. It can be used to heal small wounds, acne, fungal infections such as athlete's foot, and insect bites (Carson *et.al.*, 2006).
- **Peppermint oil** stimulates the nervous system and increases attention and concentration. It is also thought to help with indigestion and reduce certain types of headaches (Kennedy *et al.*, 2018).
- **Rosemary oil** stimulates the nervous system and is used as a remedy for exhaustion. A study has shown that mice who ingest or inhale rosemary oil became stimulated, increasing their overall movement (Kovar *et al.*, 1987).
- **Clary sage oil** is thought to ease tension and muscle cramps and can reduce acne by regulating sebum production (Ali *et al.*, 2015). It also has antimicrobial properties.

- **Eucalyptus oil** has antioxidant, anti-inflammatory and antibacterial properties (Ali *et al.*, 2015). It can be helpful for treating minor cuts and burns, along with muscle and joint pain.

Buyer beware

There is a huge range in quality of essential oils on the market because there is no governing body responsible for regulating essential oils in the United States. Some essential oils may be pure, while others contain less expensive additives. For example, the term "therapeutic grade" is sometimes included on labels, but use of this phrase is not regulated and is added to incentivize buyers to pay more.

High-quality essential oils state that the product is 100 percent essential oil with no added filler. The labels often contain the Latin name of the plant and where it was harvested. A "fragrance oil" is not a pure essential oil and has been mixed with synthetic ingredients. Lastly, high-quality oils often cost more than the imitation brands.

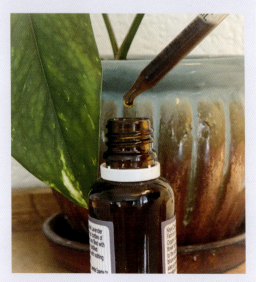

Figure 4.16 High-quality essential oil purchased from a local lavender farm.

MORE ON ESSENTIAL OILS

Essential oils have been studied in the lab. Researchers at Johns Hopkins found that essential oils from garlic cloves, myrrh trees, thyme leaves, cinnamon bark, allspice berries and cumin seeds could kill a certain type of Lyme disease bacteria in a lab dish (Feng et al., 2018). The tested essential oils worked better than standard antibiotic treatments. This finding does not suggest that essential oils should be ingested to cure Lyme disease (doing so could be toxic or fatal), but essential oils do have antibacterial properties that could possibly be formulated in a safe way to help treat conditions, such as Lyme disease, in the future.

Another group of scientists from the Instituto de Investigaciones Bioquímicas de La Plata in Argentina found that mandarin essential oil showed anticancer activity by reducing the cell growth of tumors in the lab (Manassero et al., 2013). The scientists believe that the major component of mandarin essential oil, called limonene, could someday be used for the treatment of diverse cancers.

Other studies are not so positive. Scientists from the National Institute of Environmental Health Services (NIEHS), a branch of the National Institutes of Health, studied how lavender and tea tree essential oils affected human cell lines in the lab (NIEHS, 2021). They found that both types of essential oils acted as endocrine-disrupting chemicals and altered the activity of hormones. The topical use of these essential oils has been linked with premature breast growth in girls and boys in a condition called prepubertal gynecomastia. The scientists theorize that the hormonal activity displayed by the lavender and tea tree essential oils could be causing this condition (Henley et al., 2007).

Main takeaways
- Chemosensation is the ability to sense chemicals in order to smell.
- Smell is integrated with memories within the brain.
- Aromatherapy can improve anxiety, depression, chronic pain and sleep.

TASTE

Taste is intrinsically linked with smell. Both senses rely on chemosensation to perceive chemicals in the external world. Taste is relevant to yoga and meditation because decadent foods can be incorporated into practice. Chocolate is a food of the Gods, according to the ancient Mayans, and yoga, meditation and chocolate mix quite well (Spampinato, 2022). Restorative yoga classes sometimes end with the offering of a piece of chocolate, and chocolate meditation has become popularized at some yoga studios. Chocolate meditation involves using Buddhist techniques of mindfulness to focus the attention on the act of tasting and enjoying chocolate. The goal is to become completely immersed in the experience to absorb every flavor and sensation. This results in a sensory experience, which can bring the person into the present moment to feel centered and satisfied.

Example chocolate meditation
Come to a comfortable sitting position.
Start by holding a piece of
chocolate in your hand.
Bring the chocolate to your
nose and inhale the aroma.
Let the smell seep into your body.
Let the smell activate your olfactory
neurons and send signals to your brain.
Carefully, break off a piece of
the chocolate and look at it.

Examine it, noticing the texture.
Now, slowly, bring the chocolate to your mouth and place it on your tongue.
Let it melt.
Notice the flavors as they start to activate your taste buds.
If your mind wanders, acknowledge the thought and come back to the chocolate.
Be in this present moment.
As the chocolate continues to melt, invite the sense of pleasure to fill your body.
When you're ready, carefully swallow what is left of the chocolate.
Repeat with the next piece.

Taste and the brain

The tongue is covered in lots of tiny little bumps. These bumps, called papillae, contain taste buds. Each taste bud has 50–150 specialized taste receptor cells with tiny hair-like structures called microvilli that respond to different chemicals, such as sweet, salty, sour, bitter and umami (savory, e.g. mushrooms) flavored foods (Stone *et al.*, 1995). Taste cells "live" for one to three weeks and then they regenerate. It is possible to lose function of certain taste buds, but this is usually due to damage to the nerve that connects to the individual taste bud.

Once the taste buds are activated by a chemical, the information is transported to three main cranial nerves. The first is the facial nerve (cranial nerve VII), which is connected to the front two thirds of the tongue, while the second nerve, called the glossopharyngeal nerve (cranial nerve IX), is connected to the back one third of the tongue. The third nerve involved in taste is the vagus nerve (cranial nerve X), which helps carry taste information from the back of the mouth to the brain (Figure 4.18).

Does the tongue have a map of our taste buds?

Scientists previously thought that the tongue held a unique map of taste buds, and that each area could detect different tastes. Research has shown that some areas of the tongue have taste buds that are more sensitive than other regions, but all regions of the tongue have taste buds for all flavors (Collings, 1974). In fact, the tongue has between 5,000 and 10,000 taste buds that all work harmoniously to sense sweet, salty, sour, bitter and umami.

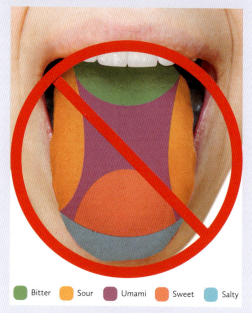

Figure 4.17 Scientists previously believed certain regions of the tongue tasted different flavors, but this has been shown to be incorrect.

Cranial nerves VII, IX and X carry information about taste to a region of the brainstem called the solitary nucleus. This group of neurons is located in the medulla and acts as a relay station for taste information. Taste information is then sent on to the thalamus for further processing before ending up in the gustatory cortex. The gustatory cortex discriminates and remembers different tastes (Rosenblum, Meiri and Dudai, 1993). Like other senses, taste information connects to the hippocampus and the amygdala to create memories of flavor preference.

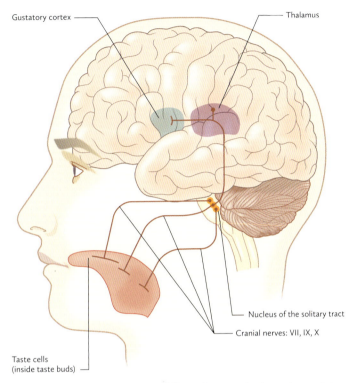

Figure 4.18 How signals about taste are transmitted from the taste buds to the gustatory cortex in the brain.

What is a supertaster?

Supertasters are people who were born with more taste buds than the average person. Some people have up to twice as many taste buds! Supertasters tend to be more sensitive to bitter flavors, such as coffee or grapefruit. It is believed that roughly 25 percent of people are supertasters (Bartoshuk et al., 1998). Supertasters tend to avoid foods that are high in fat, salt and sugar due to the strong taste, so they often have a lower risk of heart disease than normal tasters due to their healthier diets (El-Sohemy et al., 2007).

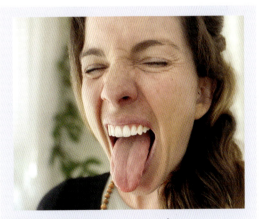

Figure 4.19 The average person has between 5,000 and 10,000 taste buds while supertasters can have twice as many!

> **Main takeaways**
> - Chocolate meditation uses Buddhist techniques of mindfulness to focus the attention on the act of tasting and enjoying chocolate.
> - All regions of the tongue have taste buds for all flavors.
> - Supertasters are people who were born with more taste buds than the average person.

TOUCH

In yoga, we touch our mats, hold onto our blocks and press our palms together in prayer. Touch is the ability to sense textures, vibration, pressures and temperatures. To perceive physical touch signals, the brain relies on receptors called **mechanoreceptors** in the skin and joints. When the body touches an object, pressure or distortion of the skin activates the mechanoreceptors. There are four main classes of mechanoreceptors that all specialize in a slightly different sensation.

> **Four main categories of mechanoreceptors**
> - **Meissner's corpuscles** are located under the skin's surface. They respond to soft touch and vibrations. These sensitive receptors help the brain decode fine touch, such as the brush of a dog's hair as they run past.
> - **Ruffini endings** are located deeper in the skin and in the connective tissue of the body. They respond when the skin is stretched and when there is an angle change in the joints.
> - **Merkel nerve endings** detect continuous pressure, like when your hands are pressed into your yoga mat during downward-facing dog.
> - **Pacinian corpuscles** are highly sensitive receptors that respond to vibration. Scientists believe they may help the brain distinguish changes in texture.

Touch sensations and the brain

Mechanoreceptors activate a chain of signals that are sent through the spinal cord to the somatosensory cortex in the brain. On their way to the brain, the signals cross the midline in the spinal cord or the brainstem. Thus, touch pathways that originate in the left side of the body are processed in the right hemisphere of the brain. Therefore, sensory information about touching a yoga block with the left hand is being processed by the right side of the brain (Figure 4.20).

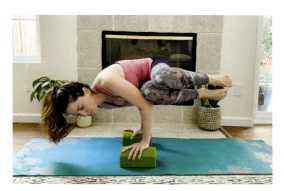

Figure 4.20 Side crow pose using blocks.

The first stop in the brain for this transmitted sensory information is the thalamus, the relay station of the brain. The thalamus then passes off relevant information to the somatosensory cortex, located in the parietal lobe, to perceive the feeling of touch (Blumenrath, 2020). The somatosensory cortex contains a topographic map that correlates to sensory regions of the body. This map has more brain area allotted to parts of the body that are most sensitive and contain the most receptors, such as the fingers and lips (Blumenrath, 2020). Figure 4.21 is a representation of the proportion of the somatosensory cortex that is devoted to each part of the body, called a **sensory homunculus**.

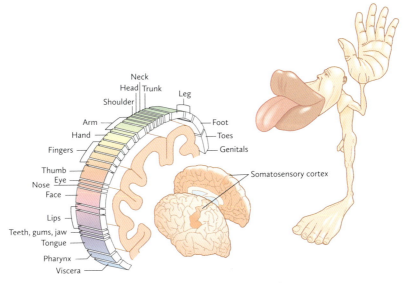

Figure 4.21 The sensory homunculus.

How does the brain deal with too many signals?

Scientists have found that successful movement involves filtering out touch signals that are less important (Conner *et al.*, 2021). For instance, when practicing yoga, we sit on a mat, while our bodies touch our clothes, and our hands reach for a water bottle. The brain is receiving a plethora of signals from touch receptors about how the body is interacting with the environment. Most of these signals do not matter, so the brain filters out the noise.

When studying the brains of mice, researchers found that neurons in a small region of the brainstem called the cuneate nucleus control how much information is passed on to other regions of the brain (Conner *et al.*, 2021).

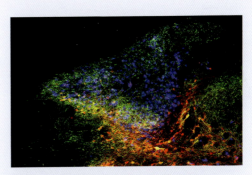

Figure 4.22 Neurons (red) in the brainstem with their axons (green) that project to the cuneate cells (blue) to transmit touch information. This circuit regulates information conveyed by touch receptors in the hands as it enters the brain.

Source: Image courtesy of the Salk Institute.

Main takeaways
- Mechanoreceptors are activated when the body touches an object.
- The four main types of mechanoreceptors include: Meissner's corpuscles, Ruffini endings, Merkel nerve endings and Pacinian corpuscles.
- The nerve pathways for touch cross at the midline, so pathways that originate in the left side of the body are processed in the right hemisphere of the brain.
- A sensory homunculus is a representation of the proportion of the somatosensory cortex that is devoted to each part of the body.

In this chapter, we have reviewed how the senses provide information to the brain and how they are often incorporated into the practice of yoga to enhance the experience in a lasting way. Throughout this chapter, we've discussed how yoga involves the senses and reviewed how the senses work. The following meditation incorporates sight, sound, smell and touch for an exercise of the senses. A piece of chocolate can also be consumed at the end to include the sense of taste.

Example meditation for the senses
Begin by coming into a comfortable sitting position.
Place your hands on your thighs with palms up or down.
Start to notice how your body feels in this position.
Notice your seat on the floor or chair.
And your hands touch your thighs.
Now, bring your attention to the sounds around you.
Fine-tune your hearing, so you can focus on the sounds far away from you.
Can you hear the birds outside or maybe even a plane?
Bring your attention to the sounds immediately around you.
Can you hear the breath move in and out of your body?
Can you hear the rustling of your clothes as your body moves with each breath?
Can you hear sounds internally, such as the gurgling of your stomach?
Now, bring your attention to your sense of smell.
What do you smell around you?
Are there any essential oils wafting in the air?
Start to notice your nervous system become more active as you search for scents.
Allow yourself to become more aware of the smells that fill your practice.
Now, bring your attention to your sense of vision.
If your eyes were closed, you can open them now.
Without moving the head, look around the room.
See the wide-open space.
And notice the objects, if any, that fill the space.
Become aware of the colors and textures around you.
Focus on the details.
And bring that same focus to the space immediately around you.
Feel how your body takes up room in this space.
Allow the eyes to close if that is available to you.
Notice the mind and allow thoughts to come and go.

> Simply acknowledge them and let them float on. As you continue to move throughout the day, think about how all of your senses are at play. Try to keep a heightened sense of the world in order to truly notice what is around you.
>
> You only get one life, so you don't want to miss a thing.
>
> Adapted from: A Meditation for Exploring Your Senses by Cara Bradley. From: https://www.mindful.org/a-meditation-for-exploring-your-senses

REFERENCES

Abhang, P.A., Gawali, B.W., & Mehrotra, S.C., 2016. Introduction to EEG- and Speech-Based Emotion Recognition. Amsterdam: Elsevier.

Alexiades, V., & Khanal, H., 2007. Multiphoton response of retinal rod photoreceptors. Sixth Mississippi State Conference on Differential Equations and Computational Simulations. *Electronic Journal of Differential Equations*, Conference 15, pp.1-9.

Ali, B., Al-Wabel, N.A., Shams, S., Ahamad, A., Khan, S.A., & Anwar, F., 2015. Essential oils used in aromatherapy: a systemic review. *Asian Pacific Journal of Tropical Biomedicine*, 5(8), pp.601-611.

Amin, A. Kumar, S.S., Rajagopalan, A., Rajan, S., Mishra, S., & Reddy, U.K., 2016. Beneficial effects of OM chanting on depression, anxiety, stress and cognition in elderly women with hypertension. *Indian Journal of Clinical Anatomy and Physiology*, 3(3), p.253.

Bao, X., Raguet L.L.G., Cole, S.M., Howard, J.D., & Gottfried, J.A., 2016. The role of piriform associative connections in odor categorization. *eLife*, 5, e13732.

Bartoshuk, L., Duffy, V.B., Lucchina, L.A., Prutkin, J., & Fast, K., 1998. PROP (6-n-propylthiouracil) supertasters and the saltiness of NaCl. *Annals of the New York Academy of Sciences*, 855, pp.793-796.

Blumenrath, S., 2020. The neuroscience of touch and pain. *BrainFacts.org*. Available at: https://www.brainfacts.org/thinking-sensing-and-behaving/touch/2020/the-neuroscience-of-touch-and-pain-013020

Bormann, J.E., Thorp, S.R., Smith, E., Glickman, M., et al., 2018. Individual treatment of posttraumatic stress disorder using mantram repetition: a randomized clinical trial. *American Journal of Psychiatry*, 175(10), pp.979-988.

Bushdid, C., Magnasco, M.O., Vosshall, L.B., & Keller, A., 2014. Humans can discriminate more than 1 trillion olfactory stimuli. *Science*, 343(6177), pp.1370-1372.

Carson, C.F., Hammer, K.A., & Riley, T.V., 2006. Melaleuca alternifolia (Tea Tree) oil: a review of antimicrobial and other medicinal properties. *Clinical Microbiology Review*, 1;19(1), pp.50-62.

Collings, V.B., 1974. Human taste response as a function of locus of stimulation on the tongue and soft palate. *Perception and Psychophysics* 16, 169-174.

Conner, J.M., Bohannon, A., Igarashi, M., Taniguchi, J., Baltar, N., & Azim, E., 2021. Modulation of tactile feedback for the execution of dexterous movement. *Science*, 374(6565), pp.316-323.

Courtiol, E., & Wilson, D.A., 2015. The olfactory thalamus: unanswered questions about the role of the mediodorsal thalamic nucleus in olfaction. *Frontiers in Neural Circuits*, 9, p.49.

Curtis, S., & Leppla, L., 2018. Instrumental activities of daily living changes in deaf and hard-of-hearing individuals after an 8-week yoga intervention. *The American Journal of Occupational Therapy*, 72(4 Supplement 1).

Devlin, K., Alshaikh, J.T., & Pantelyat, A., 2019. Music therapy and music-based interventions for movement disorders. *Current Neurology and Neuroscience Reports*, 19(11), p.83.

El-Sohemy, A., Stewart, L., Khataan, L., Fontaine-Bisson, B., et al., 2007. Nutrigenomics of taste – impact on food preferences and food production. *Forum of Nutrition*, 60, pp.176-182.

Erkkilä, J., Punkanen, M., Fachner, J., Ala-Ruona, E., et al., 2011. Individual music therapy for depression: randomised controlled trial. *British Journal of Psychiatry*, 199(2), pp.132-139.

Feng, J., Shi, W., Miklossy, J., Tauxe, G.M., McMeniman, C.J., & Zhang, Y., 2018. Identification of essential oils with strong activity against stationary phase *Borrelia burgdorferi*. *Antibiotics*, 7(4), p.89.

Geretsegger, M., Elefant, C., Mössler, K.A., & Gold, C., 2014. Music therapy for people with autism spectrum disorder. *Cochrane Database of Systematic Reviews*, CD004381.

Gheban, B.A., Rosca, I.A., & Crisan, M., 2019. The morphological and functional characteristics of the pineal gland. *Medicine and Pharmacy Reports*, 92(3), pp.226-234.

Gómez Gallego, M., & Gómez García, J., 2017. Musicoterapia en la enfermedad de Alzheimer: efectos cognitivos, psicológicos y conductuales. *Neurología*, 32(5), pp.300-308.

Gunjawate, D.R., & Ravi, R., 2021. Effect of yoga and meditation on tinnitus: a systematic review. *The Journal of Laryngology & Otology*, 135(4), pp.284-287.

Heather, S., 2007. What is sound healing? *The International Journal of Healing and Caring*, 7(3).

Henley, D.V., Lipson, N., Korach, K.S., & Bloch, C.A., 2007. Prepubertal gynecomastia linked to lavender and tea tree oils. *New England Journal of Medicine*, 356(5), pp.479–485.

Hunt, T., 2018. The hippies were right: it's all about vibrations, man! *Scientific American Blog Network*. Available at: https://blogs.scientificamerican.com/observations/the-hippies-were-right-its-all-about-vibrations-man

Jain, R., 2020. Ajna chakra: your third-eye chakra awakening. *Arhanta Yoga Blog*. Available at: https://www.arhantayoga.org/blog/ajna-chakra-your-third-eye-chakra-awakening

Kennedy, D., Okello, E., Chazot, P., Howes, M.J., et al., 2018. Volatile terpenes and brain function: Investigation of the cognitive and mood effects of Mentha × Piperita L. essential oil with in vitro properties relevant to central nervous system function. *Nutrients*, 7;10(8): pp.1029.

Kenny, M., Bernier, R., & DeMartini, C., 2005. Chant and be happy: the effects of chanting on respiratory function and general well-being in individuals diagnosed with depression. *International Journal of Yoga Therapy*, 15(1), pp.61–64.

Khalsa, D.S., Amen, D., Hanks, C., Money, N., & Newberg, A., 2009. Cerebral blood flow changes during chanting meditation. *Nuclear Medicine Communications*, 30(12), pp.956–961.

Kovar, K., Gropper, B., Friess, D., & Ammon, H.P., 1987. Blood levels of 1,8-cineole and locomotor activity of mice after inhalation and oral administration of rosemary oil. *Planta Medica*, 53(04), pp.315–318.

Malpaux, B., Migaud, M., Tricoire, H., & Chemineau, P., 2001. Biology of mammalian photoperiodism and the critical role of the pineal gland and melatonin. *Journal of Biological Rhythms*, 16(4), pp.336–347.

Manassero, C.A., Girotti, J.R., Mijailovsky, S., García de Bravo, M., & Polo, M., 2013. In vitro comparative analysis of antiproliferative activity of essential oil from mandarin peel and its principal component limonene. *Natural Product Research*, 27(16), pp.1475–1478.

Martinez, N., 2021. What you need to know about sound healing. *Mind Body Green*. Available at: https://www.mindbodygreen.com/0-17515/what-you-need-to-know-about-sound-healing.html

Melville, G.W., Chang, D., Colagiuri, B., Marshall, P.W., & Cheema, B.S., 2012. Fifteen minutes of chair-based yoga postures or guided meditation performed in the office can elicit a relaxation response. *Evidence-Based Complementary and Alternative Medicine*, 2012, 501986.

Mohanty, S., Hankey, A., Pradhan, B., & Ranjita, R., 2016. Yoga-teaching protocol adapted for children with visual impairment. *International Journal of Yoga*, 9(2), p.114.

Moore, R.Y., 1995. Neural control of the pineal gland. *Behavioural Brain Research*, 73(1–2), pp.125–130.

Moore, R.Y., Speh, J.C., & Leak, R.K., 2002. Suprachiasmatic nucleus organization. *Cell and Tissue Research*, 309(1), pp.89–98.

National Institute of Environmental Health Services (NIEHS), 2021. Essential oils. Available at: https://www.niehs.nih.gov/health/topics/agents/essential-oils/index.cfm

Nichols, D.E., 2017. N,N-dimethyltryptamine and the pineal gland: separating fact from myth. *Journal of Psychopharmacology*, 32(1), pp.30–36.

Perry, G., Polito, V., & Thompson, W., 2016. Chanting meditation improves mood and social cohesion. *Proceedings of the 14th International Conference on Music Perception and Cognition*.

Rankhambe, H., & Pande, S., 2021. Effect of "om" chanting on anxiety in bus drivers. *National Journal of Physiology, Pharmacy and Pharmacology*, 11(2), p.1.

Rolls, E., 2008. Functions of the orbitofrontal and pregenual cingulate cortex in taste, olfaction, appetite and emotion. *Acta Physiologica Hungarica*, 95(2), pp.131–164.

Rosenblum, K., Meiri, N., & Dudai, Y., 1993. Taste memory: the role of protein synthesis in gustatory cortex. *Behavioral and Neural Biology*, 59(1), pp.49–56.

Shulman, R., 2018. The basest of the senses: medical unease with the sense of smell. *Hektoen International: A Journal of Medical Humanities*, 10(2).

Simpson, F.M., Perry, G., & Thompson, W.F., 2021. Assessing vocal chanting as an online psychosocial intervention. *Frontiers in Psychology*, 12, 647632.

Siponkoski, S.T., Martínez-Molina, N., Kuusela, L., Laitinen, S., et al., 2020. Music therapy enhances executive functions and prefrontal structural neuroplasticity after traumatic brain injury: evidence from a randomized controlled trial. *Journal of Neurotrauma*, 37(4), pp.618–634.

Spampinato, C., 2022. Chocolate: food of the Gods. Available at: https://carnegiemuseums.org/magazine-archive/1997/janfeb/dept6.htm

Stone, L.M., Finger, T.E., Tam, P.P., & Tan, S.S., 1995. Taste receptor cells arise from local epithelium, not neurogenic ectoderm. *Proceedings of the National Academy of Sciences*, 92(6), pp.1916–1920.

Wilkins, R.W., Hodges, D.A., Laurienti, P.J., Steen, M., & Burdette, J.H., 2014. Network science and the effects of music preference on functional brain connectivity: From Beethoven to Eminem. *Scientific Reports*, 4, 6130.

Yong, E., 2017. The myth that humans have poor smell is nonscents. Available at: https://www.theatlantic.com/science/archive/2017/05/alls-smell-that-ends-smell/526317/

CHAPTER 5

The Origin of Movement

Yoga involves intentional movements to move into and hold various postures. This chapter will explore how the nervous system and muscles work together to coordinate complex movements. A basic understanding of how the body engages in movement will enhance our knowledge of the practice of yoga as well as our ability to improve well-being through these contemplative practices.

PART I VOLUNTARY MOVEMENT: HOW THE BRAIN CONTROLS MOTION

Scientists have been trying to decode how the nervous system generates movement for the last 150 years (Schwartz, 2016). Even simple movements like raising the arms overhead require a fully coordinated brain. The nervous system synchronizes the sequence, force, angle, direction and speed of every muscle involved in the motion.

Purposeful actions, such as lifting the arms, are initiated in the frontal lobe of the brain (Figure 5.1). A part of the frontal lobe called the **motor cortex** helps to plan, control and execute these movements. The motor cortex includes three main regions: the primary motor cortex, the premotor cortex and the supplementary motor area. Each area has a specific role in helping direct voluntary movement (Figure 5.2).

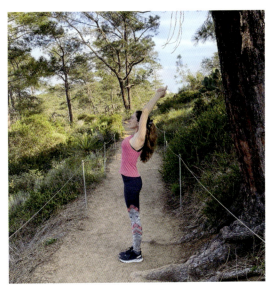

Figure 5.1 Mountain pose variation.

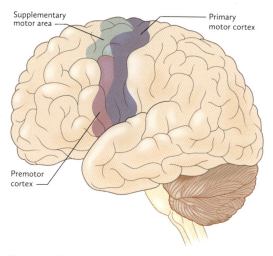

The **primary motor cortex** is the main brain region involved in the control and execution of voluntary movements (Sanes and Donoghue, 2000). This region is responsible for generating the neural impulses that activate muscles for movement. It also contains a topographic representation of the body parts involved in movement called a "motor map" or **motor homunculus** (Figure 5.3). Some parts of the body, such as the tongue and lips, take up more representative space in the brain because they involve fine-tuned movements for speaking and eating.

Figure 5.2 The key regions of the brain involved in movement.

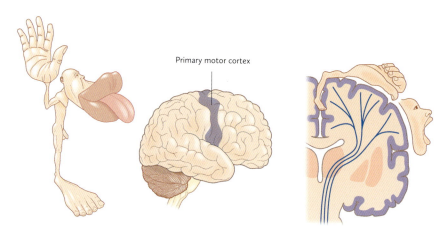

Figure 5.3 The motor homunculus.

The hands also require more representative brain area to properly function (Figure 5.4). Micro-movements in muscles of the fingers help stabilize the body in postures like downward-facing dog and crow pose. Other muscles, such as the core muscles, also aid in body stabilization, but they are limited to only less rigorously tuned movements and, thus, take up less representative space in the primary motor cortex. Think about it this way: there are over 30 muscles that make up the hands, while there are only five main abdominal muscles. The brain needs more space for these neurological connections to control the hand muscles!

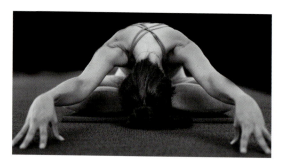

Figure 5.4 The hands take up a lot of representative space in the primary motor cortex because they involve lots of muscles to make many types of complex movements.
Source: Conscious Design on Unsplash.

Information highways for movement

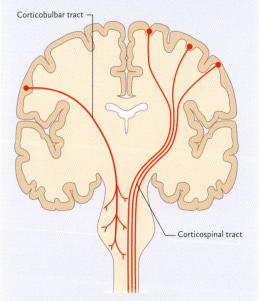

Figure 5.5 The corticobulbar tract and the corticospinal tract.

Signals traveling from the primary motor cortex are transmitted along one of two information highways: the corticospinal tract or the corticobulbar tract. The **corticospinal tract** carries signals from the brain to the spinal cord to relay information about movement of the body, while the **corticobulbar tract** sends information to the brainstem regarding movement of the head, neck and body (The Brain from Top to Bottom, 2022).

The axons in the corticospinal tract cross the body's midline at the medulla in the brainstem and continue down to the spinal cord. Thus, the right side of the brain is generally responsible for movement on the left side of the body and vice versa.

Fun fact
Giraffes have REALLY long axons in the corticospinal tract. In fact, they can easily reach 2.6 meters (8.5 feet) since they extend from the brain all the way to the end of the spinal cord (Badlangana et al., 2007).

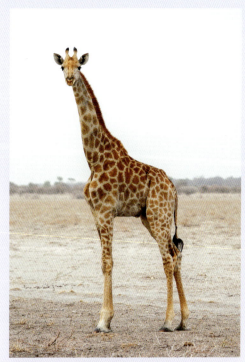

Figure 5.6 A giraffe in Botswana.
Source: Thomas Evans on Unsplash.

The **premotor cortex** sits in front of the primary motor cortex and assists in the integration of sensory and movement information to prepare a movement. The premotor cortex sends signals to the primary motor cortex, the brainstem and the spinal cord to create a plan for the body to carry out a voluntary movement.

Damage to the premotor cortex can result in a variety of seemingly odd outcomes. For instance, someone who had a stroke in their premotor cortex may not be paralyzed, but they could have difficulty performing a skilled action that could previously be performed; their brain is having trouble planning the requested action (Freund and Hummelsheim, 1985). They could also have deficits in moving their fingers and hand on the opposite side of their body or have difficulty integrating sensory information that is required to perform a movement.

The premotor cortex also contains the **supplementary motor area** (SMA), which is one of the least understood brain regions related to movement. Its neurons connect directly to the spinal cord, so it is thought to play a role in the control of movement. In addition to helping with postural control, the SMA coordinates two-handed movements (Dijkstra *et al.*, 2020; Brinkman, 1981). For instance, when bringing the hands together for a twisted chair pose, the SMA is hard at work (Figure 5.7). The SMA may also be involved with sequences of movement, such as completing a sun salutation (Verwey, Lammens and Honk, 2002). Despite advances in neuroscience, the exact role of the SMA is still unknown.

> **Main takeaways**
> - The **primary motor cortex** is the main brain region involved in the control and execution of voluntary movements. It contains a topographic representation of the body parts involved in movement called a "motor map" or "motor homunculus."
> - The **premotor cortex** assists in the integration of sensory and movement information to prepare a movement.
> - The **supplementary motor area** plays a role in the control of movement, posture, and the coordination of two-handed movement.

Other brain regions that control voluntary movement

Two additional brain regions involved in movement are the basal ganglia and the cerebellum.

THE BASAL GANGLIA

The **basal ganglia** are a group of neurons located deep within the brain that help control voluntary movement. These neurons inhibit circuits trying to initiate competing movements (Hauber, 1998). The basal ganglia help movements occur smoothly without error.

The basal ganglia do not always function properly, which can result in several different neurological conditions. Parkinson's disease occurs when the basal ganglia no longer produce enough of the neurotransmitter dopamine. People with Parkinson's often exhibit tremors and uncontrolled movements. When medications are not effective, some people with advanced Parkinson's can be treated with deep brain stimulation. This surgery involves inserting a neurostimulator that sends electrical impulses to a specific part of the basal ganglia to promote normal brain activity, allowing for better movement.

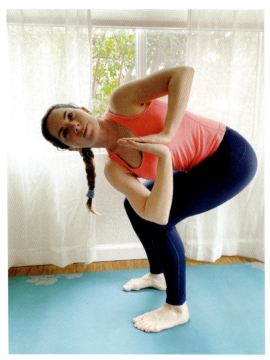

Figure 5.7 Chair pose variation with twist.

THE CEREBELLUM

The **cerebellum** helps with coordination, the timing of movement, precision, movement correction as well as motor memory (Fine, Ionita and Lohr, 2002) (Figure 5.8). In the 19th century, French physiologist Marie-Jean-Pierre Flourens discovered the cerebellum was critical for the coordination of movement by removing the cerebellums of pigeons (Kwon, 2020). He observed that the birds had balance problems once their cerebellums were absent. They walked around as if they were intoxicated. Later, doctors observed that human patients who had had cerebellar injuries, which can occur due to a tumor or stroke, acted in a similar fashion.

The cerebellum receives information about movement from multiple parts of the brain as well as receptors in the muscles, joints and tendons. It acts like an air traffic controller, directing movement related to the positioning of the limbs, the speed of the movement and any obstacles that may arise in the path ahead.

The cerebellum is also responsible for rapidly correcting movement to prevent falling. For instance, it is easy to trip over a rogue yoga block when leaving class. Instead of falling, the body quickly adjusts to correct the movement. The cerebellum is crucial for this movement correction. The cerebellum also aids with micro-corrections to promote balance in tricky postures like king dancer pose (Figure 5.9).

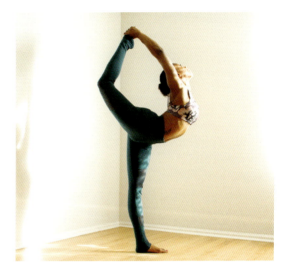

Figure 5.9 King dancer pose.
Source: Madison Lavern on Unsplash.

The cerebellum's specialized cells

The cerebellum contains specialized neurons called **Purkinje cells**. These intricately branched neurons are involved in the control of movement as well as learning. Purkinje cells regulate the rate of communication between neurons to coordinate important movements, such as moving the hands (Minai, 2014). These cells are not to be confused with Purkinje fibers located in the heart!

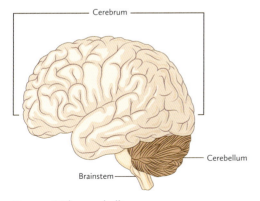

Figure 5.8 The cerebellum.

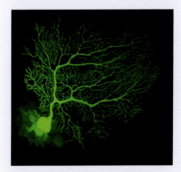

Figure 5.10 Purkinje cell from the cerebellum.
Source: Maryann Martone et al., CCDB/NCMIR/UC San Diego, CCA 3.0. From: http://www.cellimagelibrary.org/images/CCDB_3

The cerebellum also plays a role in **motor learning**. Motor learning involves learning a new movement, which can then be stored as a **motor memory**, also known as muscle memory. This type of memory allows for the recall of a specific motion or movement coordination to perform functions like riding a bike, throwing a ball, or playing an instrument years after learning how to perform the task, without much cognitive thought. Neuroscientists don't know exactly how this process works or where muscle memories are stored, but they believe the cerebellum is one of the main brain regions involved.

> **Main takeaways**
> - The **basal ganglia** are a group of neurons that help movements occur smoothly without error. Dysfunction of the basal ganglia can result in several neurological conditions, including Parkinson's disease.
> - The **cerebellum** helps with coordination, the timing of movement, precision, movement correction as well as motor memory. It contains specialized cells called Purkinje cells.

> **Sun salutations and the cerebellum**
> To celebrate a new yoga studio opening, practitioners are sometimes invited to participate in a ceremonial practice of 108 sun salutations. The number 108 is sacred and thought to represent the wholeness of existence (Yoga Journal, 2021). When practicing such repetitive movements, muscle memory kicks in and guides the body through the practice. The muscle memory of a sun salutation allows the practitioner to focus on the breath instead of where to place a hand or foot. The ability to glide through a sun salutation without much thought is largely due to the cerebellum.

Signals from the brain to the body

Although the brain directs most movements, it is the **motor neurons** that make it all happen. These specialized neurons extend from the brain or spinal cord to individual muscle fibers of a muscle to provide instructions about which muscles to move and how to move them.

Motor neurons transfer instructions to muscle fibers at the **neuromuscular junction** (Figure 5.12). Here, electrical signals trigger the release of the neurotransmitter acetylcholine, among other substances. Acetylcholine then travels across the synapse and binds to receptors on the muscle, which causes the muscle to contract, enabling movement.

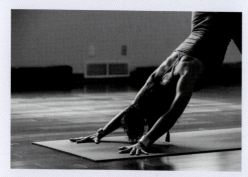

Figure 5.11 Downward-facing dog.
Source: Ginny Rose Stewart on Unsplash.

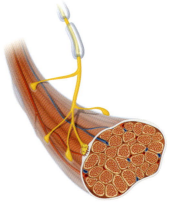

Figure 5.12 The neuromuscular junction.

The sciatic nerve

The longest and largest nerve in the body is the **sciatic nerve**. The sciatic nerve branches from the lower back into the hips and travels down the legs branching into other nerves, which continue to the toes. It contains motor neurons that help the muscles in the legs and feet move, as well as sensory neurons to send signals about sensations of the legs and feet to the brain. In a tall person, the axons of the sciatic nerve can exceed one meter (3 feet) in length (Muzio and Cascella, 2021). At its thickest point, the sciatic nerve is about as thick as your thumb!

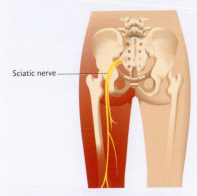

Figure 5.13 The sciatic nerve extends from the lower back to below the knee where it branches into other nerves that travel to the toes.

The sciatic nerve can sometimes become pinched or inflamed in a condition called sciatica. Sciatica often causes pain that radiates from the lower back down the leg and can lead to issues with movement of the leg and foot. It can be caused by a herniated disk; however, nearly 70 percent of all sciatica cases are caused by the piriformis muscle of the hip compressing the nerve due to tightness (Filler et al., 2005).

Yoga can help to relieve symptoms of sciatica caused by an overtight piriformis. It's important to not aggressively stretch this muscle though, as this can aggravate symptoms. Below are three postures that can help to lengthen and relax the piriformis muscle to reduce pain and discomfort.

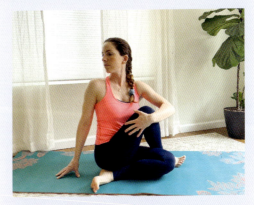

Figure 5.14 Simple seated twist.

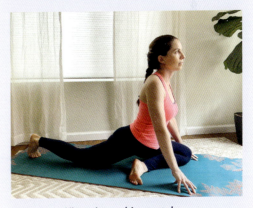

Figure 5.15 King pigeon hip stretch.

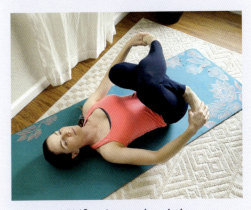

Figure 5.16 Piriformis stretch variation.

PART II INVOLUNTARY MOVEMENT: NO BRAIN REQUIRED

Doctors often use a soft rubber hammer to test the knee jerk **reflex**. This rapid movement is automatic and does not require any cognitive thought. In fact, this movement doesn't involve the brain at all.

Instead, sensory receptors in the knee perceive the impact of the hammer (which stretches the tendon) and send a signal to a **sensory neuron**, which is a nerve cell that detects and responds to the environment. The sensory neuron then transmits this information to the spinal cord where a motor neuron receives the signal and, in turn, contracts the muscle, bypassing the brain altogether (Figure 5.17).

Reflexes are a survival mechanism. For instance, the withdrawal reflex can quickly remove a hand from a burning pot, and the startle reflex enables us to leap out of the way of a potential hazard.

> **Main takeaways**
> - **Motor neurons** transmit information from the brain or spinal cord to regulate activity in muscles for movement.
> - The **neuromuscular junction** is where motor neurons transfer instructions about movement to muscle fibers.
> - The **sciatic nerve** is the longest nerve in the body, and it helps the muscles in the legs and feet move as well as feel sensations. It can easily become pinched or inflamed in a condition called sciatica.
> - A **reflex** is a rapid, automatic movement that does not involve the brain.

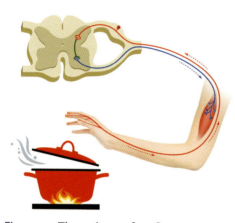

Figure 5.17 The pathway of a reflex.

PART III PROPRIOCEPTION

Imagine practicing yoga with your eyes closed. Even without vision, the body can create the shapes and movements of different yoga postures. The ability to be aware of your body's position and movement is called **proprioception**.

Proprioception relies on three main sensory systems. The first are specialized receptors located in the muscles, joints and tendons that send signals to the brain about body position. The balance system, also called the vestibular system, in the inner ear relays information about rotation, acceleration, gravity and position. And although proprioception can occur without sight, the visual sensory system is helpful for sending visual cues about body position. These three systems work together to provide the brain with an understanding of where the body is in space and how it is moving.

The brain receives signals from these three sensory systems and sends instructions back out to the muscles to coordinate movement. For example, the ability to balance requires lots of micro-adjustments, which rely heavily on signals from the cerebellum and the brainstem.

Proprioception can occur both consciously and unconsciously. Conscious proprioception is used to facilitate complex movements, movements that require concentration and thought to complete, such as doing a backbend. Unconscious proprioception is important for coordinating less complex movements, like maintaining posture and walking (Johnson *et al.*, 2008). Unconscious proprioception can occur quickly to help coordinate the body.

Many yoga postures rely on the proprioceptive system to create the shapes and movements with the body. Researchers have found that practicing yoga can improve proprioception and balance in those with neurological disorders as well as the visually impaired (Cherup *et al.*, 2020; Mohanty, Pradhan and Nagathna, 2014).

Proprioceptive receptors

Located throughout the muscles, **muscle spindles** are proprioceptive receptors that detect changes in muscle length (how stretched out the muscle is) and the speed at which the muscle length is changing (Matthews, 1964). Muscle spindles pass along this information to sensory neurons, which send signals to the central nervous system about muscle movement.

Within the tendons and joints are proprioceptive receptors called **golgi tendon organs** and **joint receptors**, respectively. Golgi tendon organs sense information about muscle tension, which is a measure of exertion, while joint receptors provide information about joint position.

The balance system

There are also exceptionally accurate sensors located in the inner ear that receive information about balance and spatial orientation. Knowing which way is up or down seems like a simple task, but it is quite complicated (Figure 5.18).

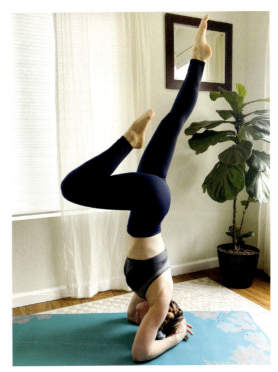

Figure 5.18 Balancing upside-down requires multiple sensory systems working together but relies heavily on the vestibular system, which senses spatial orientation and gravity.

Although the inner ear helps with hearing, it also plays a critical role in decoding spatial orientation as part of the **vestibular system**, also known as the "balance center" or "balance system." The vestibular system primarily helps us detect head movement. It also aids in providing the brain with information about head position and orientation to maintain balance and posture as well as stabilize the head during movement.

The vestibular system contains numerous structures, but the two main ones are located in the vestibular labyrinth and include the semicircular canals and otolith organs. There are three **semicircular canals** that contain fluid with tiny hair cells (Figure 5.19). Each canal is oriented in a different plane to detect one of three types of rotational head movement: nodding up and down, shaking side to side and tilting left and right (Figures 5.20–5.22).

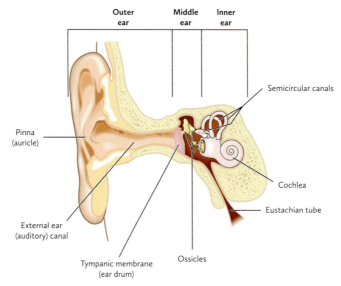

Figure 5.19 Semicircular canals within the ear.

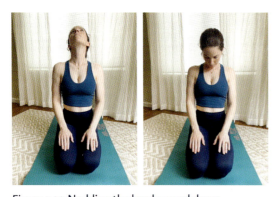

Figure 5.20 Nodding the head up and down.

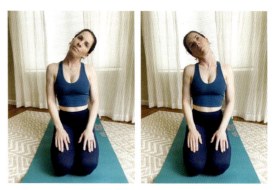

Figure 5.22 Tilting left and right.

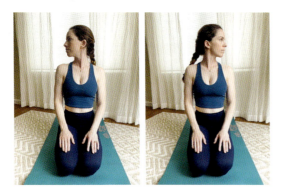

Figure 5.21 Shaking side to side.

When the head changes direction, the fluid called endolymph in the semicircular canals shifts, which signals to the hair cells that there is movement in a certain direction. The hair cells then relay this information to the vestibular nerve (a branch of the vestibulocochlear cranial nerve), which sends signals to the brain about movement and orientation.

The inner ears also contain small structures called **otolith organs** that help us sense forward and backward movements (linear acceleration) as well as gravity. They work very similarly to how the semicircular canals detect movement, involving fluid and hair cells. Both the otolith organs and the semicircular canals are necessary for the brain to understand body position.

Comparing the otolith organs with the semicircular canals

Otoliths detect linear acceleration, which is a change in speed (either increasing or decreasing) without a change in direction. Linear acceleration occurs when traveling in a straight line, like when traveling in a car and hitting the gas to avoid running a red light.

The semicircular canals detect angular acceleration, which is when there is a change in speed as well as a change in direction at the same time. Angular acceleration occurs when riding a roller coaster when it takes a 360-degree roll. The semicircular canals have three main loops that detect movement in three planes, which enables them to detect angular acceleration of the head.

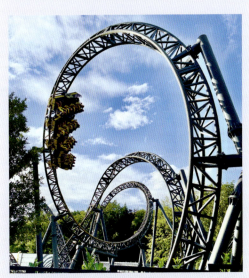

Figure 5.23 The semicircular canals detect angular acceleration, like what is experienced when riding a roller coaster.
Source: Jonny Gios on Unsplash.

The semicircular canals and the otolith organs enable the vestibular system to know where the head is located in space and how it is moving. The vestibular system can then use this knowledge to influence eye movements to hold the gaze steady. Gaze stabilization, such as concentrating on a focal point, is often used during yoga, especially to avoid falling during balance postures or when transitioning from one position to another. The vestibular system is especially important for standing balance control, and dysfunction of this system can lead to issues with stability (van Kordelaar *et al.*, 2018).

Why do people get motion sickness?

Motion sickness occurs when the vestibular system and the visual system disagree. This can occur when sitting in a boat on a windy day. The motion of the ocean waves causes the fluid in the inner ears to shift, and the hair cells signal to the brain that the body is in motion. However, the body is sitting in the boat and not moving, so the muscle spindle receptors tell the brain that the body is not in motion. This conflict in signaling to the brain leads to nausea.

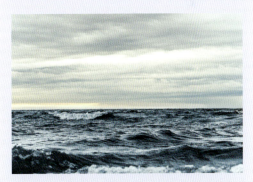

Figure 5.24 People often experience motion sickness when travelling over rough water.
Source: Ant Rozetsky on Unsplash.

Main takeaways
- **Proprioception** is awareness of the position and movement of the body.
- Proprioceptor receptors include muscles spindles, golgi tendon organs and joint receptors.
- The **vestibular system** is the body's balance center. It helps the brain detect head movement and aids in gaze stability.
- The **semicircular canals** each detect a different type of rotational head movement: nodding up and down, shaking side to side and tilting left and right.
- The **otolith organs** sense forward and backward movements as well as gravity.
- Practicing yoga can improve proprioception and balance.

Proprioception and yoga

Just like practicing a skill, proprioceptive abilities can be cultivated with repetition. Yoga can help to develop self-awareness of the body, improving the ability to know where the body is in space, control the muscles, and balance (Cherup *et al.*, 2020). One study found that practicing tree pose for two minutes a day increased the static and dynamic balance of older women (Solakoglu *et al.*, 2021). Another study showed that practicing Hatha yoga twice a week for 12 weeks could improve balance in those with Parkinson's disease, a condition that often alters one's ability to balance (Elangovan *et al.*, 2020). Taken together, these findings suggest that balance can improve with yoga practice, including in older individuals and those with neurological disorders.

Another way to increase proprioceptive abilities is to practice yoga with the eyes shut. Basic postures can become quite difficult when the visual system is turned off, forcing the brain to rely on other proprioceptive systems more heavily. It can also be informative to film yourself practicing a sequence with your eyes closed.

Then you can review the footage to see if you were moving your body as you thought.

Below is an example yoga routine for working on body awareness and balance. To make a posture more accessible, try gazing at a certain point on the floor or wall. If you would like more of a challenge, try closing your eyes. You can also slow down the transitions between postures to focus on muscle control and coordination.

EXAMPLE YOGA SEQUENCE FOR PROPRIOCEPTION AND BALANCE

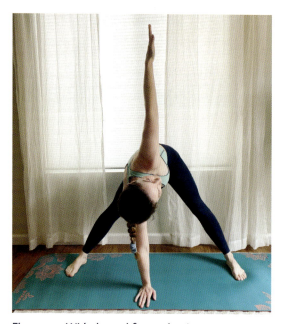
Figure 5.25 Wide-legged forward twist.

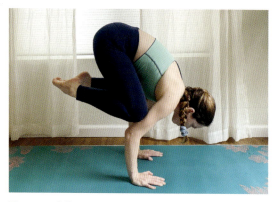
Figure 5.26 Crow pose.

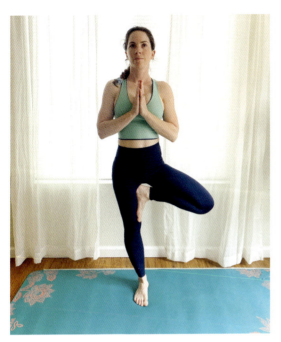

Figure 5.27 Tree pose.

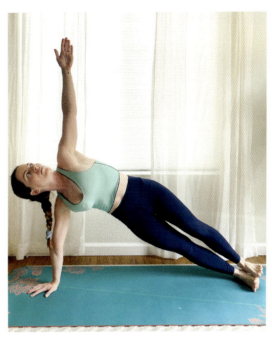

Figure 5.29 Side plank variation. The top leg can also be lifted for an added balance challenge.

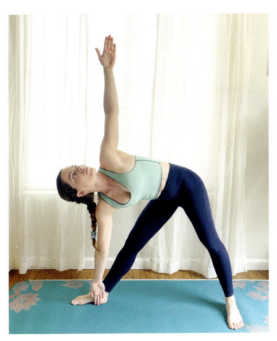

Figure 5.28 Triangle pose.

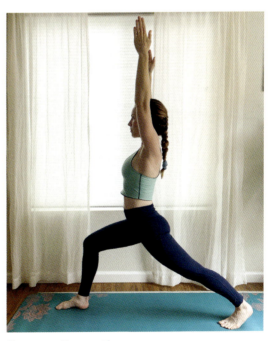

Figure 5.30 Crescent lunge.

REFERENCES

Badlangana, N.L., Bhagwandin, A., Fuxe, K., & Manger, P.R., et al., 2007. Observations on the giraffe central nervous system related to the corticospinal tract, motor cortex and spinal cord: what difference does a long neck make? *Neuroscience*, 148(2), pp.522–534.

Brinkman, C., 1981. Lesions in supplementary motor area interfere with a monkey's performance of a bimanual coordination task. *Neuroscience Letters*, 27(3), pp.267–270.

Cherup, N.P., Strand, K.L., Lucchi, L., Wooten, S.V., Luca, C., & Signorile, J.F., 2020. Yoga meditation enhances proprioception and balance in individuals diagnosed with Parkinson's disease. *Perceptual and Motor Skills*, 128(1), pp.304–323.

Dijkstra, B.W., Bekkers, E.M.J., Gilat, M., Rond, V.D., Hardwick, R.M., & Nieuwboer, A., 2020. Functional neuroimaging of human postural control: a systematic review with meta-analysis. *Neuroscience & Biobehavioral Reviews*, 115, pp.351–362.

Elangovan, N., Cheung, C., Mahnan, A., Wyman, J.F., Tuite, P., & Konczak, J., 2020. Hatha yoga training improves standing balance but not gait in Parkinson's disease. *Sports Medicine and Health Science*, 2(2), pp.80–88.

Filler, A.G., Haynes, J., Jordan, S.E., Prager, J., et al., 2005. Sciatica of nondisc origin and piriformis syndrome: diagnosis by magnetic resonance neurography and interventional magnetic resonance imaging with outcome study of resulting treatment. *Journal of Neurosurgery: Spine*, 2(2), pp.99–115.

Fine, E.J., Ionita, C.C., & Lohr, L., 2002. The history of the development of the cerebellar examination. *Seminars in Neurology*, 22(4), pp.375–384.

Freund, H.-J., & Hummelsheim, H., 1985. Lesions of premotor cortex in man. *Brain*, 108(3), pp.697–733.

Hauber, W., 1998. Involvement of basal ganglia transmitter systems in movement initiation. *Progress in Neurobiology*, 56(5), pp.507–540.

Johnson, E.O., Babis, G.C., Soultanis, K.C., & Soucacos, P.N., 2008. Functional neuroanatomy of proprioception. *Journal of Surgical Orthopaedic Advances*, 17(3), pp.159–165.

Kwon, D., 2020. The mysterious, multifaceted cerebellum. *BrainFacts.org*. Available at: https://www.brainfacts.org/brain-anatomy-and-function/anatomy/2020/the-mysterious-multifaceted-cerebellum-120320

Matthews, P.B., 1964. Muscle spindles and their motor control. *Physiological Reviews*, 44(2), pp.219–288.

Minai, M., 2014. Purkinje cells. *The Embryo Project Encyclopedia*. Available at: https://embryo.asu.edu/pages/purkinje-cells

Mohanty, S., Pradhan, B., & Nagathna, R., 2014. The effect of yoga practice on proprioception in congenitally blind students. *British Journal of Visual Impairment*, 32(2), pp.124–135.

Muzio, M.R., & Cascella, M., 2021. Histology, Axon. In: StatPearls [Internet]. Treasure Island (FL): StatPearls Publishing; 2022 Jan-. Available at: https://www.ncbi.nlm.nih.gov/books/NBK554388/

Sanes, J.N., & Donoghue, J.P., 2000. Plasticity and primary motor cortex. *Annual Review of Neuroscience*, 23(1), pp.393–415.

Schwartz, A.B., 2016. Movement: how the brain communicates with the world. *Cell*, 164(6), pp.1122–1135.

Solakoglu, O., Dogruoz Karatekin, B., Yumusakhuylu, Y., Mesci, E., & Icagasioglu, A., 2021. The effect of yoga asana "Vrksasana (tree pose)" on balance in patients with postmenopausal osteoporosis. *American Journal of Physical Medicine & Rehabilitation*, 101(3), pp.255–261.

The Brain from Top to Bottom, 2022. The Axons Entering and Leaving the Motor Cortex. McGill University. Available at: https://thebrain.mcgill.ca/flash/i/i_06/i_06_cl/i_06_cl_mou/i_06_cl_mou.html

van Kordelaar, J., Pasma, J.H., Cenciarini, M., Schouten, A.C., Kooij, H.V.D., & Maurer, C., 2018. The reliance on vestibular information during standing balance control decreases with severity of vestibular dysfunction. *Frontiers in Neurology*, 9, p.371.

Verwey, W.B., Lammens, R., & Honk, J. van, 2002. On the role of the SMA in the discrete sequence production task: a TMS study. *Neuropsychologia*, 40(8), pp.1268–1276.

Yoga Journal, 2021. What's so sacred about the number 108? *Yoga Journal*. Available at: https://www.yogajournal.com/practice/yoga-sequences/the-number-108

CHAPTER 6

The Neurophysiology of the Breath

Breathing is a life-sustaining action for all animals on earth, and it is a critical aspect of contemplative practices like yoga or meditation.

Today, scientists are still discovering how breathing can impact heart rate, digestion, the immune system and even the brain.

PHYSIOLOGY OF THE INHALATION AND EXHALATION

The inhalation can oxygenate the muscles, slow the heartbeat, stabilize blood pressure and reduce stress. Inhaling air, which contains roughly 80 percent nitrogen and 20 percent oxygen, initiates a cascade of reactions that affect every system in the body.

During the inhalation, air travels from the mouth or nose down the pharynx, commonly known as the throat. The air then flows into the trachea, also known as the windpipe (Figure 6.1). The trachea is divided into two relatively large air passages called the right bronchus and left bronchus, which connect to the right lung and left lung, respectively. The right lung has three sections (called lobes) and is slightly larger than the left lung, which only has two sections. The bronchi then divide into even smaller bronchioles within the lungs, like a tree trunk dividing into branches over and over again. The bronchioles end in tiny air sacs called alveoli, which transfer oxygen from inhaled air into the bloodstream (Figure 6.2). The oxygenated blood is then pumped throughout the body to provide oxygen to cells.

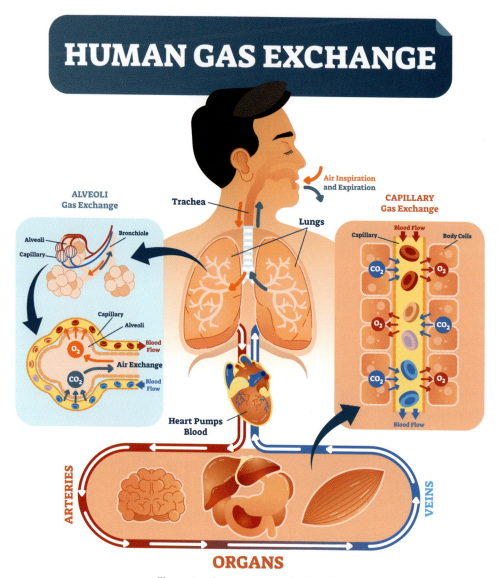

Figure 6.1 The anatomy of the breath.

As the cell uses oxygen, it produces carbon dioxide as waste. Carbon dioxide is carried in the bloodstream to the lungs so it can be removed during the exhalation.

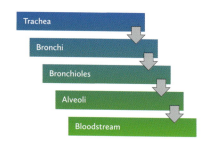

Figure 6.2 The anatomical flow of the breath.

THE IMPORTANCE OF THE NOSE

The phrase "breathe in through the nose and out through the mouth" is frequently used in yoga and meditation classes, although the science behind this cue is often left out. Humans are designed to breathe through their noses. Young babies inhale using the nose to nurse and breathe at the same time, and athletes inhale through the nose to slow down heart rate and improve athletic performance.

The nose controls the temperature of the inhaled air by warming it during the breath. The lungs are sensitive to colder temperatures, which make them constrict and take shallower breaths. For example, when running outside on a crisp day, it can feel difficult to take a deep breath. To compensate for this reaction, the nose warms the air before it enters the lungs, so that the lungs can properly expand to take in oxygen.

The nose also regulates the humidity of the air entering the lungs. Nasal breathing adds moisture to the air to prevent a sore throat and dry mouth. During the winter months, people who mouth-breathe may experience a sore throat because the air is not being humidified by the nose. The nose is also filled with tiny little hairs called cilia that trap debris and toxins to prevent them from getting into the lungs.

Lastly, the nose conveys the sense of smell through the olfactory nerve. The ability to smell aids in detecting harmful toxins, such as smoke from a burning building. During a yoga or meditation class, the instructor may burn incense or spray essential oils, which can elevate the practice by adding the dimension of scent.

The nose knows

The nose is full of erectile tissue; the same type of tissue as in the genitals (Figure 6.3). Erectile tissue in the nose has an important regulatory role. By expanding and shrinking, the erectile tissue can alter the diameter of the nostril, which changes the speed and volume of the airflow coming into the body (Ng, Ramsey and Corey, 1999). In turn, this regulates the warming and humidification of the air.

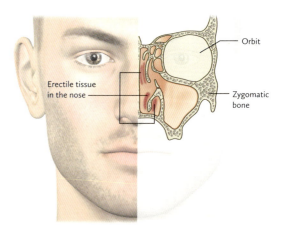

Figure 6.3 Erectile tissue in the nose.
Adapted from: https://www.researchgate.net/figure/The-location-of-the-erectile-tissue-inside-the-nasal-cavity_fig10_229079961, CC BY 2.5.

This erectile tissue in the nose swells and settles throughout the day in a cyclical manner (Kahana-Zweig et al., 2016). This allows for greater airflow in one nostril at a time, shifting from left to right and back again. An ancient yoga text called the *Shiva Swarodaya* describes the flow of this phenomenon of nasal cycles in the form of energy (Telles and Naveen, 2008; Rai, 2012). In the text, the breath is considered the cosmic life force, and people who practice Swara yoga focus on different types of breathing. There are three main types of breathing in Swara yoga which include breathing through: 1) the left nostril, 2) the right nostril and 3) both nostrils. Each type of breathing is aligned with the cycles of the moon, as the nostrils naturally rotate through creating their own natural rhythms (Saraswati, 1982).

There haven't been any research studies on Swara yoga specifically, but scientists do know that the nostrils pulse throughout the day. The nasal cycle has been documented using structural

MRI (Kahana-Zweig et al., 2016). One nostril may swell for 25 minutes to a few hours and then relax as the opposite nostril starts to swell. The result is an alternating, partial congestion and decongestion that occurs unconsciously throughout the day.

These nasal cycles are likely driven by the autonomic nervous system. While the sympathetic nervous system is associated with constricting blood vessels in one nostril, the parasympathetic nervous system dilates blood vessels in the other nostril. Slower breathing can create a more powerful cycle between the two nostrils with each having more robust swelling and then decompression (Kahana-Zweig et al., 2016).

The nasal cycle is also associated with health and disease. For example, during sickness or stress, the nose becomes inflamed. These states can cause the nasal cycle to speed up, switching from left to right more quickly to better control things like temperature as well as chemicals that can affect the brain (Nestor, 2021). One case study of a schizophrenic female also showed an imbalance between breathing through her left and right nostril (Shannahoff-Khalsa and Golshan, 2015). When the scientists introduced exercises to correct this imbalance, her hallucinations decreased. Thus, there could be a link between the nasal cycle and some disease states. However, the sample size of one limits the conclusions that can be drawn and more research needs to be conducted.

> **Main takeaways**
> - Breathing through the nose is important in yoga and meditation to slow down the heart rate and increase oxygenation.
> - The nose controls the air temperature of inhaled air as well as the humidity.
> - The nose also contains erectile tissue that expands and shrinks throughout the day to naturally regulate the flow of the breath.

THE BREATH AND THE BRAIN

The average human takes 25,000 breaths every day (Gross, 2020). Breathing occurs unconsciously or with conscious thought depending on the level of attention to the breath. Most of the time, breathing is not a conscious endeavor. The body naturally inhales and exhales air. But how does the body regulate this activity?

It all comes down to sophisticated machinery in the blood vessels and a tiny breathing center in the brainstem. The body senses the levels of oxygen, carbon dioxide and pH using specialized sensors in our carotid arteries in the neck and the aortic arch of the heart called **chemoreceptors** (Prabhakar, 2000) (Figure 6.4).

When the levels of carbon dioxide in the blood increase too much, the chemoreceptors send signals to a part of the brainstem called the medulla that the body needs more oxygen. The medulla instructs the breathing muscles, the muscles that wrap around the rib cage and the diaphragm, to contract and relax to bring fresh air into the lungs. These muscles allow for the inhale (an inspiration) as well as the exhale (an expiration). The medulla also maintains the breathing rhythm to breathe at a regular pace (Ikeda et al., 2016). If the body is not receiving enough oxygen, then the chemoreceptors will send signals to the medulla to tell the lungs to breathe more frequently.

When oxygen levels are low in the body, the medulla can also send signals to the heart, instructing it to pump faster to circulate oxygenated blood. The communication between the medulla, the lungs and the heart is primarily through the vagus nerve, the main nerve of the parasympathetic nervous system.

Scientists believe that the breath may stimulate the vagus nerve through respiratory vagal nerve stimulation (Gerritsen and Band, 2018). The autonomic nervous system relies on the balance between the sympathetic nervous system and the parasympathetic nervous system. While the sympathetic nervous system can raise heart rate, blood pressure and respiration rate, the parasympathetic nervous system can lower these factors and increase digestion. Specifically, the vagus nerve can be suppressed during inhalation and activated during exhalation and the slowing of the breath rate (Chang et al., 2015; Gerritsen and Band, 2018). Thus, slow, controlled deep breathing fills the body with oxygen and signals to the brain that it is time to relax.

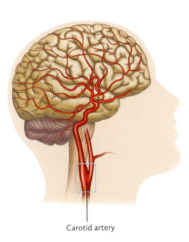

Carotid artery

Figure 6.4 The carotid artery contains chemoreceptors that can sense blood oxygenation levels. Each side of the neck contains a carotid artery that carries blood to the neck and head. If you place two fingers on the side of your neck you can feel the pulse of your blood from your heart traveling through your carotid arteries.

Main takeaways
- **Chemoreceptors** in the carotid arteries send signals to the medulla in the brainstem about blood oxygenation levels. If the body is not receiving enough oxygen, then the medulla will send signals to the lungs to breathe more frequently.
- The communication between the medulla, the lungs and the heart is primarily through the vagus nerve, the main nerve of the parasympathetic nervous system.
- Slow, controlled deep breathing fills the body with oxygen and promotes relaxation.

The breath and mood

The breath can be a powerful tool for altering mood. For example, long, deep breaths bring forth feelings of calm and relaxation, while a more forceful breath may energize the body. For centuries, humans have been using slow, controlled breathing to promote a calm state of mind and reduce arousal during times of stress, like during a panic attack. Yet, until recently, researchers did not know *how* the breath affected states of mind.

Researchers at Stanford University stumbled upon the connection between the breath and the mind by accident while examining the neurons in the brainstems of mice (Yackle et al., 2017). The scientists were interested in a group of neurons in the medulla that control respiratory rhythms called the pre-Bötzinger complex, and they wanted to know more about the specific roles of neurons in this region. To learn more, the scientists destroyed a subpopulation of neurons and observed if there was any change in behavior in mice.

The researchers found that mice without this subpopulation of pre-Bötzinger complex neurons could still breathe with a normal rhythm, but they were unusually calm and relaxed. The scientists were stumped. Why would destroying breathing neurons in the brainstem make the mice calmer?

They had stumbled upon the link between breathing, stress and emotion. This subpopulation of pre-Bötzinger complex neurons sends signals to the locus coeruleus, which produces the neurotransmitter norepinephrine. The release of norepinephrine drives the stress response, arousal, fear and anxiety. Thus, these breathing neurons regulate the balance between calm and arousal behaviors. Breathing techniques likely work by altering the activity of the pre-Bötzinger complex to regulate the activity of the locus coeruleus, which alters mood.

Breathing through stress, pain and anxiety

During stress, the rate of respiration increases. Under immediate stress, like running away from a lion, breathing quickly is not a problem. However, people with chronic stress or anxiety tend to breathe more frequent, shallow breaths over an extended period, continuously activating the sympathetic nervous system. The sympathetic nervous system, in turn, releases more stress hormones like cortisol that can damage cells.

The breath can be used to our advantage. By practicing slow, controlled breathing it is possible to train the body to trigger the parasympathetic nervous system, instead of the sympathetic nervous system.

> **Tip for breathing through stress**
> If you're stressed, one way to hack your autonomic nervous system is to simply take an extended breath in through the nose. This action sends a direct signal to your brain that your body is in recovery mode – time to relax.

Scientists from the Technical University of Munich in Germany also showed that mindful attention to the breath can relieve stress and negative emotions (Doll et al., 2016). In the study, 26 participants were trained in mindful attention to the breath for two weeks. They then entered an MRI machine where they practiced attention to the breath and were presented with stress-inducing images, while the scientists examined which areas of their brains became activated. The researchers found that attentional focus on the breath activated the prefrontal cortex and reduced activity in the amygdala. This pattern of brain activity produced calming emotions.

Focusing on the breath draws the mind away from worries. Mindfulness trains the brain to focus on the present moment, instead of allowing the mind to shift into a place of anxiety and rumination. Practitioners can harness this knowledge to calm the mind by practicing breathing exercises and meditation.

Breathing is also connected to the experience of pain and anxiety. Intense psychological pain can induce hyperventilation, a state when breathing becomes rapid and shallow. Scientists from the Salk Institute for Biological Studies were interested in uncovering which group of neurons in the mouse brain were responsible for coordinating breathing with psychological pain, along with negative emotions such as anxiety (Liu et al., 2021). They focused their study on a group of neurons called the pontine respiratory group (PRG) located in the brainstem. The PRG neurons are not involved with generating respiratory rhythms (that is the job of the respiratory group in the medulla), but rather control the rate and pattern of breathing.

Within the PRG is a smaller group of neurons called the parabrachial nucleus. Activating the parabrachial nucleus has been shown to both increase and slow down breathing. The authors wanted to see if a subpopulation of neurons in the parabrachial nucleus, called *Oprm1*-expressing neurons, coordinated breathing with pain and emotions, as is seen in pain-induced hyperventilation. Using a variety of scientific techniques, the scientists mapped, monitored and manipulated the neural circuit in mice to see how the breathing rate was affected.

They found that the brain circuit regulating breathing rate involved two populations of *Oprm1*-expressing neurons both found in the parabrachial nucleus. The first group called the shell neurons were connected to the breathing center of the brain (the pre-Bötzinger complex), while the second group of neurons called the core neurons connected to pain and emotional centers (the amygdala) (Figure 6.5). When both of these populations of neurons were stimulated, the mice showed increased psychological pain and negative emotional behaviors.

In an interview with *NPR*, the lead scientist Sung Han stated that the two circuits were intrinsically linked together (Hamilton, 2021). "If that's also true in people, it would help explain the mysterious connection between breathing and emotion, which has puzzled scientists for centuries."

The scientists note that breathing and negative emotions do not always influence each other. For example, during exercise, breathing rate is increased and emotional states can improve. In this case, and others like it, these *Oprm1*-expressing neurons may not be involved or have a different sort of involvement. This is one of the first studies to show how breathing is connected, on a molecular and mechanistic level, with pain and emotions, such as anxiety.

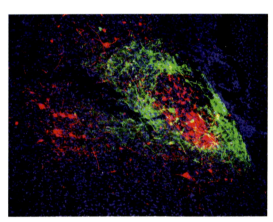

Figure 6.5 Shell neurons (green) that project to the breathing center and core neurons (red) that project to the pain/emotion center.

Source: Image courtesy of the Salk Institute. From: https://www.salk.edu/news-release/pain-and-anxiety-impact-breathing-on-a-cellular-level

Main takeaways
- Groups of neurons in the medulla connect breathing with stress, pain and emotion.
- Slow, controlled breathing can be used to trigger the parasympathetic nervous system to promote relaxation.
- Mindful breathing can relieve stress and negative emotions by activating the prefrontal cortex and reducing activity in the amygdala.

CONSCIOUS CONTROL OF THE BREATH

Humans can control their breath through conscious thought. Controlled yogic breathing is called **pranayama**, and it is one of the eight limbs of traditional yoga (Rain *et al.*, 2021). Pranayama has been mentioned in some of the earliest yogic texts, such as the *Bhagavad Gita* and *The Yoga Sutras of Patanjali*.

The word "pranayama" is composed of two Sanskrit terms, "prana" and "yama." Prana is defined as the vital life force that keeps us all alive, while yama refers to control or restraint. Thus, pranayama is collectively thought of as techniques for breath control. Many contemplative practices, such as yoga and meditation, incorporate pranayama to improve mental and physical health.

Exercises with conscious control of the breath can have both immediate and long-term effects. For example, one study showed that deep breathing exercises improve blood oxygen levels in people with lung injuries (Malik and Tassadaq, 2019). When a person exercises, carbon dioxide is produced, and the blood starts to become acidic. Breathing counters this acidity by exhaling carbon dioxide and bringing more oxygen into the bloodstream through the lungs.

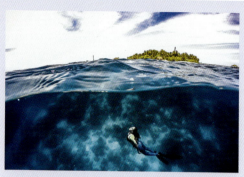

Figure 6.6 Free divers can alter their physiology over time, allowing them to hold their breath longer than the average adult.
Source: Sebastian Pena Lambarri on Unsplash.

> **Fun fact**
> One of the most extreme examples of breath practice comes in the form of free diving. Free divers can hold their breath for over five minutes as they dive, perfectly focused and calm, over a hundred meters under water. The Austrian free diver Herbert Nitsch currently holds the Guinness World Record after free diving 253 meters (830 feet) off the coast of Santorini, Greece.
>
> Free divers have developed what is known as a "diving response," which involves breathing very slowly and the constriction of the blood vessels throughout the body (Tetzlaff *et al.*, 2021). The body also synergistically activates both the sympathetic and parasympathetic nervous systems, while increasing the release of catecholamines, reducing the heart rate and redistributing blood to vital organs (Tetzlaff *et al.*, 2021).
>
> Professional free divers work on developing this diving response to alter their physiology. One way that they do this is through repeated oxygen deprivation, called apnea training. This training also increases their ability to hold air in their lungs (called lung capacity), and some free divers have a lung capacity of 10 liters or more, nearly double that of an average adult.

Types of controlled breathing

Many different types of breath control are practiced around the world. The following are a few common ones that are used in yoga and meditation research.

Mindful breathing is a breathing technique that focuses the attention on the breath. When practicing mindful breathing, the practitioner breathes in a way that feels natural to them. The practitioner simply acknowledges the breath and notices its qualities. Mindful breathing can be practiced with the eyes open or closed depending on the type of practice and the comfort level of the practitioner.

Deep breathing is a technique used to invite relaxation throughout the body. It can also help to relieve stress and anxiety. This practice can be performed in any comfortable position, such as lying down, sitting or even standing. One form of deep breathing involves taking a long, deep breath and holding that breath for a few seconds at a time, before releasing it. Another form of deep breathing is when the practitioner extends either the inhale, exhale or both for a period of time. Deep breathing activates the parasympathetic nervous system and calming centers in the brain by decreasing respiration rate and increasing the length of the breath.

Diaphragmatic breathing, also known as belly breathing, is a technique that activates the diaphragm to draw air into the lungs. There are a few ways to practice diaphragmatic breathing, but one of the easiest and simplest methods is to lie on your back with your legs bent and feet flat on the floor. Place one hand on the belly, below the rib cage, to feel the movement of the diaphragm. Take a smooth inhale and feel the belly expand, pushing into the hands. Then exhale the breath, trying to push the belly down towards the floor, engaging the transverse abdominal muscles. Once the practice becomes easy on the floor, it can be practiced in a chair or even while standing or walking.

Alternate nostril breathing is a technique that relies on breathing through one nostril at a time using the fingers to open and close each side in an alternating fashion. Alternate nostril breathing is similar to the Swara yogic breathing that was discussed earlier in the chapter, but the two forms of pranayama have different origins. This practice is best avoided when feeling congested or sick, as this will result in difficulty breathing. Begin by coming into a comfortable seated position. Welcome a clearing breath and then take the right thumb and press against the right nostril, closing the passageway. Take an inhale, allowing the air to enter only through the left nostril. Then close the left nostril and allow the exhale to leave through the right nostril. Continue the breathing practice, alternating between the left and right nostrils for the inhale and exhale.

What does the science say? The benefits of controlled breathing

The science of the breath is an area of research that is gaining a lot of attention in the neuroscience community due to the direct effect of the breath on the mind. Some scientists have even argued that the rhythmic activity of the breath could regulate brain activity (Heck *et al.*, 2017). Below is a summary of the latest research on the different types of breathing exercises.

MINDFUL BREATHING

Mindful breathing exercises are associated with better cognition, emotion regulation, mood, working memory and attention (Eisenbeck, Luciano and Valdivia-Salas, 2018; Schöne *et al.*, 2018). Practicing mindful breathing could also alter brain networks. Researchers from Osnabrück University in Germany and Liverpool John Moores University in the UK used an electroencephalogram (EEG) to examine differences in brain waves of mindfulness meditators in comparison with a muscle relaxation group when performing an attention task (Schöne *et al.*, 2018). They found that mindful breath awareness led to refinements in brain networks involved in attention. The mindful breathers may be using their brains more efficiently when focusing on a task.

A review of 22 studies conducted by researchers at Suffolk University in Massachusetts examined the neurological underpinnings of mindfulness practices (Falcone and Jerram, 2018). Across the studies, mindfulness practices were related to activity in the frontal regions, anterior cingulate and insula. The authors state that their findings are consistent with how mindful breathing can impact cognition and learning regions of the brain (Falcone and Jerram, 2018).

DEEP BREATHING

Deep breathing is a powerful form of breath control. Even a single session of deep, slow breathing has been shown to reduce stress and anxiety as well as increase parasympathetic activity (Magnon, Dutheil and Vallet, 2021).

Deep breathing exercises affect brain activity, mood and behavior. In a review of the literature, researchers at the University of Pisa in Italy examined 15 published articles and found that the prefrontal, motor and parietal cortices all showed increased activity during a task in subjects who practiced deep breathing (Zaccaro *et al.*, 2018). Additionally, participants across many studies reported improved relaxation, alertness and comfort with reduced symptoms of anxiety, anger, arousal and confusion.

Researchers have also found that the effects of slow, deep breathing on the body are substantial and immediate. In a large study of 80 participants, scientists from Nepal Medical College in Kathmandu asked participants to breathe in for a count of four seconds and then exhale for a count of six seconds for five continuous minutes (Manandhar and Pramanik, 2019). After performing the breathing exercise, the participants showed a trend towards decreased blood pressure and quicker reaction times, indicating greater alertness and faster information processing.

Additional studies have shown that other types of slow breathing exercises can have immediate effects as well. For example, slow bhastrika pranayama (respiratory rate: 6 breaths/min) and bhramari pranayama (respiratory rate: 3 breaths/min) decreased blood pressure, with a slight decrease in heart rate after five minutes of practice (Pramanik *et al.*, 2009; Pramanik, Prajapati and Pudasaini, 2010). Sukha pranayama (respiratory rate: 6 breaths/min) was also found to significantly decrease heart rate, systolic blood pressure and arterial pressure in hypertensive patients after five minutes (Bhavanani, Sanjay and Madanmohan, 2011).

> **Deep breathing exercise**
> Take an inhalation for a count of four.
> Now, slowly exhale for a count of four.
> Inhale for a count of four.
> Exhale for a count of six.
> Inhale for a count of four.
> Exhale for a count of eight.
> Repeat three times.
> Take a few moments for self-reflection.
> Notice the change in your body
> and your overall mental state.

DIAPHRAGMATIC BREATHING

An international group of researchers examined the effect of diaphragmatic breathing on attention, cognition, mood and stress (Ma *et al.*, 2017). In the study, 40 participants were assigned to either the diaphragmatic breathing condition (20 people) or the control condition (20 people). The people in the diaphragmatic breathing group received 20 sessions of breathing training over eight weeks using a real-time feedback device. They averaged four breaths per minute when performing the diaphragmatic breathing.

The scientists found that participants who had performed the diaphragmatic breathing had improved mood and attention versus before the breathing practice. The breathing group also had significantly lower cortisol levels, a measure of the stress response, after the intervention. The control group showed none of these changes. These findings suggest that diaphragmatic breathing could improve psychological and physiological states, which has important implications for health promotion and maintenance.

ALTERNATE NOSTRIL BREATHING

Although not entirely backed by science, many alternate nostril breathing practitioners believe that breathing through the right nostril activates the sympathetic nervous system, while breathing through the left nostril activates the parasympathetic nervous system. In this sense, breathing through the right nostril acts as a gas pedal, increasing blood pressure, heart rate, body temperature and cortisol levels (Kumari, Kalaivani and Pal, 2019; Nestor, 2021), whereas breathing through the left nostril acts as a brake, decreasing these physiological reactions.

Alternate nostril breathing may also be a helpful strategy for reducing stress and anxiety. Scientists from Kasturba Medical College in India studied how alternate nostril breathing right before public speaking reduced anxiety (Kamath, Urval and Shenoy, 2017). In the study, the researchers had 15 medical students practice 15 minutes of alternate nostril breathing, while an additional 15 medical students sat quietly in a room. Both groups were then instructed to prepare a four-minute speech in two minutes. They found that the breathing group showed a trend towards lower levels of anxiety.

Some scientists have argued that in addition to activating different nervous systems, alternate nostril breathing can also impact different sides of the brain. Researchers from S-VYASA Yoga University in India looked at the effect of right and left nostril breathing on the two hemispheres of the brain (Bhargav, Singh and Srinivasan, 2016). The scientists measured the blood oxygen levels in the brains of 32 male participants using a near-infrared system, a brain imaging method that measures the light absorbance in order to estimate oxygenated blood as an indirect measure of brain activity. They found that right nostril breathing increased blood oxygenation and blood volume in the left hemisphere of the brain (specifically the prefrontal cortex). Conversely, they found that left nostril breathing showed a trend towards decreasing blood oxygenation in the right hemisphere.

Although the authors argue that their findings support the idea of uni-nostril breathing to oxygenate separate sides of the brain, their results are inconclusive at best, given that the left nostril breathing showed no significant results. Thus, whether or not alternate nostril breathing influences hemispheric brain activity remains a controversial research topic that neuroscientists must explore further in the future.

CULTIVATING RESILIENCE WITH THE BREATH

Breathing exercises can be used to train the body to be more resilient by dampening the body's reaction to stressful situations. Slow, deep breathing activates the parasympathetic nervous system and signals to the body to produce fewer stress hormones during periods of stress.

The term "relaxation response" was coined by Harvard researcher Herbert Benson in the 1970s, and it has been used in academic research ever since (Benson and Proctor, 2011). Throughout his work, Benson has shown that meditation can counter the effects of stress. Additionally, Benson, along with researchers from Massachusetts General Hospital and Beth Israel Deaconess Medical Center, found that the relaxation response can also produce immediate changes in gene expression related to inflammation, immune functioning, metabolism and longevity (Bhasin et al., 2013). The mind can be used to change the body. Thus, breathing can be a powerful tool for cultivating resilience on a molecular level.

But it wasn't until fairly recently that doctors and scientists started taking the whole body into account when considering human health. The idea that the body and mind are separate entities, a construct called dualism, was popularized by French philosopher René Descartes. Descartes' dualism was especially prevalent in medicine, where the body was often treated separately from the mind. However, more and more research now demonstrates how our mind and body are linked on the molecular and cellular level. Although Descartes was a brilliant thinker, dualism may have been his greatest error (Damasio, 2008).

Today, scientists around the world are exploring the many ways in which the mind and body are connected, and one area of focus is how the mind and body connection can synergistically help build resilience. Scientists from Ohio State University examined the effects of an online mind–body skills training in health professionals (Kemper and Khirallah, 2015). The large study consisted of 513 participants who were either dietitians, nurses, physicians, social workers, clinical trainees or health researchers. The scientists found that mindfulness-based stress reduction techniques improved mindfulness, resilience and empathy across all participants.

> **Resilience meditation**
>
> Come into a comfortable position.
> Start to notice your thoughts,
> and the state of your mind.
> Do you feel stressed? Relaxed?
> Tired? Energized?
> Notice how the body feels.
> Feel if there is any tension.
> Take a deep breath in and out,
> letting the tension release.
> When the body relaxes, our
> mind can also relax.
> Roll both shoulders down and back.
> Now, bring the right ear down
> to the right shoulder.
> Release. And bring the left ear
> down to the left shoulder.
> Start to roll the chin from left to right,
> releasing any tension in the neck.
> Come back to center and check in
> with the state of your mind again.
> It may feel a little quieter and calmer.
> Wherever you are, start to
> stretch your body.
> Make yourself as long as possible.
> Stress contracts the body, so we
> are counteracting those effects.
> Take a long, deep breath and hold
> it while contracting the body.
> Hold the body tight for 5 seconds.
> Then release the breath and the body.
> Feel the new state of the body and mind.
>
> *Adapted from: Resilience Meditation by Emma Seppälä, author of the book The Happiness Track. From: https://www.youtube.com/watch?v=SNc-nElydr8*

Main takeaways
- **Pranayama** refers to a group of techniques for breath control.
- Some of the most common forms of controlled breathing studied in research include mindful breathing, deep breathing, diaphragmatic breathing, and alternate nostril breathing. All of these practices have been shown to have different benefits for mental and physical health.
- Harvard researcher Herbert Benson has shown that slow, deep breathing can trigger the relaxation response, which produces immediate changes in gene expression related to inflammation, immune functioning, metabolism and longevity.

REFERENCES

Benson, H., & Proctor, W., 2011. *Relaxation Revolution: The Science and Genetics of Mind Body Healing*. New York; London; Toronto; Sydney: Scribner.

Bhargav, H., Singh, K., & Srinivasan, T.M., 2016. Effect of uninostril yoga breathing on brain hemodynamics: a functional near-infrared spectroscopy study. *International Journal of Yoga*, 9(1), p.12.

Bhasin, M.K., Dusek, J.A., Chang, B., Joseph, M.G., *et al.*, 2013. Relaxation response induces temporal transcriptome changes in energy metabolism, insulin secretion and inflammatory pathways. *PLoS ONE*, 8(5), e62817.

Bhavanani, A.B., Sanjay, Z., & Madanmohan, 2011. Immediate effect of sukha pranayama on cardiovascular variables in patients of hypertension. *International Journal of Yoga Therapy*, 21(1), pp.73–76.

Chang, R.B, Strochlic, D.E., Williams, E.K., Umans, B.D., & Liberles, S.D., 2015. Vagal sensory neuron subtypes that differentially control breathing. *Cell*, 161(3), pp.622–633.

Damasio, A., 2008. *Descartes' Error: Emotion, Reason and the Human Brain*. London: Vintage Digital.

Doll, A., Hölzel, B.K., Bratec, S.M., Boucard, C.C., et al., 2016. Mindful attention to breath regulates emotions via increased amygdala–prefrontal cortex connectivity. *NeuroImage*, 134, pp.305–313.

Eisenbeck, N., Luciano, C., & Valdivia-Salas, S., 2018. Effects of a focused breathing mindfulness exercise on attention, memory, and mood: the importance of task characteristics. *Behaviour Change*, 35(1), pp.54–70.

Falcone, G., & Jerram, M., 2018. Brain activity in mindfulness depends on experience: a meta-analysis of FMRI studies. *Mindfulness*, 9(5), pp.1319–1329.

Gerritsen, R.J., & Band, G.P., 2018. Breath of life: the respiratory vagal stimulation model of contemplative activity. *Frontiers in Human Neuroscience*, 12, p.397.

Gross, T., 2020. Deep breaths: how breathing affects sleep, anxiety & resilience. Available at: https://www.npr.org/2020/05/27/863395357/deep-breaths-how-breathing-affects-sleep-anxiety-resilience

Hamilton, J., 2021. Studies into how pain and breathing are connected could lead to safer pain drugs. *NPR Illinois*. Available at: https://www.nprillinois.org/2021-12-17/studies-into-how-pain-and-breathing-are-connected-could-lead-to-safer-pain-drugs

Heck, D.H., McAfee, S.S., Liu, Y., Babajani-Feremi, A., et al., 2017. Breathing as a fundamental rhythm of brain function. *Frontiers in Neural Circuits*, 10, p.115.

Ikeda, K., Kawakami, K., Onimaru, H., Okada, Y., et al., 2016. The respiratory control mechanisms in the brainstem and spinal cord: integrative views of the neuroanatomy and neurophysiology. *The Journal of Physiological Sciences*, 67(1), pp.45–62.

Kahana-Zweig, R., Geva-Sagiv, M., Weissbrod, A., & Secundo, L., et al., 2016. Measuring and characterizing the human nasal cycle. *PLoS ONE*, 11(10), e0162918.

Kamath, A., Urval, R.P., & Shenoy, A.K., 2017. Effect of alternate nostril breathing exercise on experimentally induced anxiety in healthy volunteers using the simulated public speaking model: a randomized controlled pilot study. *BioMed Research International*, 2017, pp.1–7.

Kemper, K.J., & Khirallah, M., 2015. Acute effects of online mind–body skills training on resilience, mindfulness, and empathy. *Journal of Evidence-Based Complementary & Alternative Medicine*, 20(4), pp.247–253.

Kumari, M.J., Kalaivani, S., & Pal, G.K., 2019. Effect of alternate nostril breathing exercise on blood pressure, heart rate, and rate pressure product among patients with hypertension in Jipmer, Puducherry. *Journal of Education and Health Promotion*, 8(1), p.145.

Liu, S. Ye, M., Pao, G.M., Song, S.M., et al., 2021. Divergent brainstem opioidergic pathways that coordinate breathing with pain and emotions. *Neuron*, 110(5), pp. 857–873.e9.

Ma, X., Yue, Z., Gong, Z., Zhang, H., et al., 2017. The effect of diaphragmatic breathing on attention, negative affect and stress in healthy adults. *Frontiers in Psychology*, 8, p.874.

Magnon, V., Dutheil, F., & Vallet, G.T., 2021. Benefits from one session of deep and slow breathing on vagal tone and anxiety in young and older adults. *Scientific Reports*, 11(1), p.19267.

Malik, S.S. & Tassadaq, N., 2019. Effectiveness of deep breathing exercises and incentive spirometry on arterial blood gases in second degree inhalation burn patients. *Journal of the College of Physicians and Surgeons Pakistan*, 29(10), pp. 954–957.

Manandhar, S.A., & Pramanik, T., 2019. Immediate effect of slow deep breathing exercise on blood pressure and reaction time. *Mymensingh Medical Journal*, 28(4), pp.925–929.

Nestor, J., 2021. *Breath: The New Science of a Lost Art*. London: Penguin Life.

Ng, B.A., Ramsey, R.G., & Corey, J.P., 1999. The distribution of nasal erectile mucosa as visualized by magnetic resonance imaging. *Ear, Nose & Throat Journal*, 78(3), pp.159–166.

Prabhakar, N.R., 2000. Oxygen sensing by the carotid body chemoreceptors. *Journal of Applied Physiology*, 88(6), pp.2287–2295.

Pramanik, T., Sharma, H.O., Mishra, S., Mishra, A., Prajapati, R., & Singh, S., 2009. Immediate effect of slow pace bhastrika pranayama on blood pressure and heart rate. *The Journal of Alternative and Complementary Medicine*, 15(3), pp.293–295.

Pramanik, T., Prajapati, R., & Pudasaini, B., 2010. Immediate effect of Buteyko breathing and Bhramari Pranayama on blood pressure, heart rate and oxygen saturation in hypertensive patients: a comparative study. *Nepal Medical College Journal*, 12(3), pp.154–157.

Rai, R.K., 2012. *Shiva Svarodaya*. Varanasi, India: Prachya Prakashan.

Rain, M., Subramaniam, B., Avti, P., Mahajan, P., & Anand, A., 2021. Can yogic breathing techniques like Simha Kriya and Isha Kriya regulate COVID-19-related stress? *Frontiers in Psychology*, 12, p.635816.

Saraswati, S.M., 1982. Swara yoga – Part 4: Rhythmic flow of the Swara. Available at: http://www.yogamag.net/archives/1980s/1982/8204/8204sw4.html

Schöne, B., Gruber, T., Graetz, S., Bernhof, M., & Malinowski, P., 2018. Mindful breath awareness meditation facilitates efficiency gains in brain networks: a steady-state visually evoked potentials study. *Scientific Reports*, 8(1), p.13687.

Shannahoff-Khalsa, D., & Golshan, S., 2015. Nasal cycle dominance and hallucinations in an adult schizophrenic female. *Psychiatry Research*, 226(1), pp.289–294.

Telles, S., & Naveen, K.V., 2008. Voluntary breath regulation in yoga: its relevance and physiological effects. *Biofeedback*, 36(2), pp.70–73.

Tetzlaff, K., Lemaitre, F., Burgstahler, C., Luetkens, J., & Eichhorn, L., 2021. Going to extremes of lung physiology – deep breath-hold diving. *Frontiers in Physiology*, 12, p.710429.

Yackle, K., Schwarz, L.A., Kam, K., Sorokin, J.M., *et al.*, 2017. Breathing control center neurons that promote arousal in mice. *Science*, 355(6332), pp.1411–1415.

Zaccaro, A., Piarulli, A., Laurino, M., Garbella. E., *et al.*, 2018. How breath-control can change your life: a systematic review on psycho-physiological correlates of slow breathing. *Frontiers in Human Neuroscience*, 12, p.353.

CHAPTER 7

Meditation and the Brain

Meditation has been used for thousands of years to calm and quiet the mind (Figure 7.1). Although meditation has its roots in ancient India, it has become a popular practice in the West. Numerous research studies demonstrate the wide range of benefits from practicing meditation, such as reducing symptoms of stress, anxiety, depression and pain while improving well-being and cognition. This chapter will explore the science of meditation and discuss how the brain is involved in this contemplative practice. Not surprisingly, as we remain on the frontier of understanding the brain, the studies of the brain and meditation point in a variety of interesting directions.

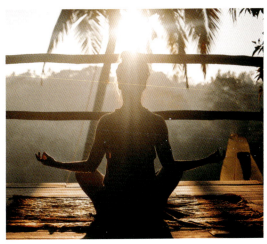

Figure 7.1 Meditation offers many health benefits.
Source: Jared Rice on Unsplash.

THE FOUR CATEGORIES OF MEDITATION IN RESEARCH

To better study and compare the effects of meditative practices, researchers have characterized meditation styles into four main categories: 1) focused-attention meditation, 2) mantra recitation meditation, 3) loving-kindness meditation and 4) open-monitoring meditation (Fox *et al.*, 2016).

Focused-attention meditation requires a focus or concentration on a specific object or theme, such as the breath or a visualization, while disengaging from the wandering mind.

The breath is often used as a target of focus. When the mind starts to fill with thoughts, the practitioner can refocus their attention back to the target. Focused-attention meditation develops the skill of attentional control, which is critical for functioning and thriving in everyday life. Some examples of focused-attention meditation include Zen meditation, candle gazing and breath meditations, during which the focus is on the breath (Brandmeyer, Delorme and Wahbeh, 2019).

Shamatha meditation is also a style of focused-attention meditation. Shamatha means "peaceful abiding" or "tranquility," and this type of mindfulness meditation stems from Buddhist tradition (Owens, 2021). During Shamatha meditation, the practitioner first focuses on an object or the breath, and then, with experience, they meditate being mindful of the present moment while cultivating the acceptance of thoughts.

> **Example Shamatha meditation**
> Come to a comfortable seated position.
> Start to become aware of the breath.
> Notice as the breath enters
> and exits the body.
> As thoughts enter your mind, let them
> go and come back to the breath.
> Stay here, practicing this method.
> Start to come back to the breath,
> focusing on the inhale and exhale.
> Feel the breath get sucked in and
> then pushed out of the body.
> Feel the cyclical nature of the breath.
> Once you're ready, invite the breath
> to pause in the body for a few seconds
> before releasing it for an exhalation.
> The breath becomes an inhalation,
> a hold, and an exhalation.
> As you inhale try to make the sound "om."
> As you hold the breath chant "ah."
> And as you exhale, sound out "hung."
> These sacred syllables help to
> bring even more awareness to your
> practice and purify the mind.
>
> *Adapted with permission from: How to Practice Shamatha Meditation by Lama Rod Owens. From: https://www.lionsroar.com/how-to-practice-shamatha*

Mantra recitation meditation involves the repeated recitation of a sound, word or phrase either out loud or in one's head to promote focus and intention. This type of meditation is similar to a focused-attention meditation except that the object of focus is verbal rather than a bodily sensation, such as breathing. Additionally, because the focus of mantra recitation meditation is on verbal cues, instead of bodily sensations, it is likely this style of meditation uses different brain regions than other styles of meditation (Fox *et al.*, 2016).

Mantra meditation may also involve the practitioner moving mala beads through their fingers as they recite their mantra. Ideally, the mantra is not too long, so it can be easily repeated. With practice, the vibration of the sounds is thought to provide happiness and peace by feeling the presence of what is traditionally called *shakti* – the subtle force within us that brings about awareness (Moran, 2018).

One of the most common mantras practiced around the world is the chanting of the word "Om," which is said to be the sound of the creation of the universe. It is believed to contain every vibration that has ever existed or will exist in the future (Moran, 2018).

> **Example mantra meditation**
> Come to a comfortable seated position.
> Close your eyes if that is accessible to you.
> And start to focus on the breath.
> Once the body has relaxed, start
> to repeat your mantra.
> Repeat the mantra slowly and steadily,
> concentrating on the sounds of the words.
> Find a natural rhythm with
> your voice and the breath.
> You can repeat part of your mantra on the
> inhale and the other part on the exhale.
> Or if it's short, then it can
> be repeated on both.

> Once you feel comfortable and confident
> with verbalizing your mantra, start
> to recite it internally, to yourself.
> If thoughts start to invade your mind,
> simply come back to your mantra.
> Come back to the sound.
> Allow the mantra to float away
> and come back to your breath.
> Now, connect with yourself.
> How are you feeling?

Loving-kindness and compassion meditation centers on cultivating love, kindness and compassion towards others and oneself using a variety of mental techniques. These types of meditation can shift behavioral and affective patterns towards more positive states (Brandmeyer, Delorme and Wahbeh, 2019).

Typically, when learning this style of meditation, love and kindness are first cultivated for someone you love. In the second stage, love and kindness are sent to yourself. In the third stage, positive feelings are sent to someone you might have difficulty sending loving thoughts to. In the final stage, the feelings of love and kindness can be expanded to all living things. Of course, there are many variations on how to practice loving-kindness meditation. Some people prefer to start with cultivating positive feelings towards themselves and then expand outward. It depends on which feelings are most accessible to the practitioner.

Below is an example of an introductory loving-kindness meditation in which the meditator first focuses on cultivating love and kindness for someone they love. After, they transmit those feelings towards a neutral person.

It is not necessary to go through all the stages during every meditation. Instead, it can be helpful to start slow and ease into developing these positive feelings.

> **Example loving-kindness meditation**
> Come into a comfortable position and close your eyes.
> Take a deep breath in and breathe out.
> Start to think of a person close
> to you who loves you.
> Imagine that person sending you love.
> They wish you to be safe and happy.
> Feel the warmth coming from that person.
> You start to become filled with
> this warmth and love.
> Begin to send this warmth and
> love back to that person.
> Wish them safety and happiness.
> Now, start to think of an acquaintance,
> someone you don't know very well.
> Choose someone who you have
> no strong feelings towards.
> Start to send warmth and
> love to this person.
> Wish them safety and happiness.
> Now come back to the breath,
> focusing on the inhale and exhale.
> Take a deep breath in and let it go.
> Flutter the eyes open and come
> back into the present moment.

In **open monitoring meditation**, the attention is brought to the present moment without a focus on a specific object (Brandmeyer, Delorme and Wahbeh, 2019). The practitioner allows thoughts and sensations to be observed without judgment. These thoughts and sensations can be positive, neutral or even negative in nature. Mental content is neither contemplated nor suppressed. Examples of this category of meditation include mindfulness meditation and Vipassana meditation.

Mindfulness meditation is a general term that can include multiple styles of meditation. At a basic level, mindfulness is the ability to be fully present in the current moment. This state includes being aware of thoughts, emotions and sensations that your body and mind are experiencing. During mindfulness meditation, the practitioner is asked to experience the moment without judgment. Instead, they are encouraged to cultivate curiosity, warmth and kindness about the human experience.

Mindfulness meditation became popularized in the Western world through researchers such as John Kabat-Zinn, Herbert Benson and Richard Davidson, along with Vietnamese Buddhist monk Thích Nhất Hạnh (Harrington and Dunne, 2015). Mindfulness is now practiced by millions of people and incorporated into a large variety of therapeutic programs. In fact, mindfulness-based interventions, such as Zinn's Mindfulness-Based Stress Reduction (MBSR) program, have been used to help treat multiple conditions, including anxiety, chronic pain and sleep disturbances (Goldin and Gross, 2010; Rosenzweig et al., 2010; Carlson and Garland, 2005).

> **Example mindfulness meditation**
> Come into a comfortable position,
> either sitting or lying down.
> Place your palms facing up if
> that is accessible to you.
> Start to bring your awareness to your face.
> Notice if there is any tension in your
> forehead, your eyes, or your cheeks.
> Release this tension and feel
> those muscles start to relax.
> Now, bring your focus to your jaw.
> Release your jaw from clenching.
> Feel those muscles relax.
> Bring your attention to your neck,
> both the front and the back.
> Breathe into the muscles, inviting release.
> Continue this technique of scanning each
> part of your body until you reach your toes.
> Stay aware of any thoughts, emotions or sensations that arise.

Vipassana meditation is one of the oldest forms of Buddhist mindfulness meditation (Chiesa, 2010). It uses mindful breathing and body awareness to focus on whatever arises in the present moment, including thoughts and emotions, in a nonjudgmental way instead of trying to control the experience. The goal is to gain a clear understanding of reality. Vipassana meditation is also known as insight meditation or mindfulness (Emavardhana and Tori, 1997).

> **Example Vipassana meditation**
> Come to a comfortable seated position.
> Close your eyes and start
> to breathe naturally.
> Focus on the natural rhythm of the breath.
> Notice how this breath feels as it
> moves in and out of the body.
> Become aware of each inhale and exhale.
> Start to notice if you have any
> thoughts, feelings or sensations.
> Observe them without judgment and let them pass.
> If you become distracted,
> return to the breath.
> Stay with the breath and continue to
> observe thoughts, feelings or sensations.
> And then let them go.

Zen meditation is another type of open-monitoring meditation. It is a seated Buddhist practice that is thought to have originated in China during the Tang dynasty. It involves an open, undirected awareness of the present moment where the body, breath and mind are acknowledged as one whole being. The long-term benefits of Zen meditation include stress reduction, improved cognition and changes in brain structures related to attentional processing (Pagnoni and Cekic, 2007).

> **Example Zen/Zazen meditation**
> Come to a comfortable seated position, keeping the back straight and centered. Allow the breath to flow in and out effortlessly. If you can, close the mouth and allow the breath to enter and leave through the nose. The gaze of the eyes can lower to a point almost a meter (a few feet) in front of you. The focus now comes to the breath. Release any tension in the body by feeling the breath relax the self. Completely experience the breath. You can start to count the inhales and exhales until you reach ten. Then repeat. If your mind begins to wander, simply come back to the breath. This action of returning to the breath is developing mindfulness. Try to be patient with yourself. Mindfulness will come with practice.

THE NEUROANATOMY OF MEDITATION

Over the last three decades, neuroscientists have examined how meditation can change brain structure as well as brain function. Although there are multiple categories and styles of meditation, the term "meditation" is sometimes used loosely in research papers. Due to the lack of differentiation between styles, it is often difficult to discern which type of meditation is even being studied! Despite this setback, numerous studies have been conducted on how meditation affects brain structure and function. Many of these preliminary studies are limited in sample size and/or lack a control group, which builds a foundation for future research.

> **Could one style of meditation be more beneficial than another?**
> It could be! But we don't know. There is a large gap in the literature around testing and comparing the different styles of meditation. Thus, little is currently known about whether one type of meditation is more beneficial or leads to more brain changes than another.

MEDITATION AFFECTS BRAIN STRUCTURE

The brain can adapt and change with experiences, learning and behavior. These brain changes can occur at the cellular level and affect everything from gray matter (neuronal cell bodies) to white matter (neuronal axons) of different brain regions. The invention of neuroimaging has allowed researchers to look inside the brains of meditators, exploring what brain anatomy is unique to this contemplative practice.

One of the first neuroimaging studies of meditators was conducted by researchers at Massachusetts General Hospital, MIT and Harvard Medical School in 2005. They found that people with extensive insight meditation experience had thicker cortices than the control group, including the prefrontal cortex and the insula (Lazar et al., 2005). As explained in an earlier chapter, the prefrontal cortex is involved in cognitive control, decision making and attention, whereas the insula is responsible for self-awareness and

interoception, the ability to sense the internal state of the body.

The scientists also found that older, experienced meditators showed less cortical thinning (which can be caused by the death of neurons) in these areas compared with the control group. Their findings suggest that a regular meditation practice could be neuroprotective and promote brain health.

This study, like many that came after it, was hindered by a small sample size (20 participants in this case). One of the main limitations in neuroimaging research is that magnetic resonance imaging machines are extremely expensive to operate. Studies with small sample sizes can still be useful, but they should be considered preliminary and in need of replication with larger sample sizes to confirm results.

Review of current studies: gray matter and white matter differences

Reviews and meta-analyses of this literature are important tools for understanding a field constrained by small sample sizes. In one such study, researchers from the University of British Columbia analyzed 21 neuroanatomy studies with roughly 300 total participants (Fox *et al.*, 2014). The studies reviewed were diverse and included meditation styles such as insight, Zen, mindfulness-based stress reduction and others. About half of the studies analyzed failed to list the type of meditation studied or included participants that practiced multiple styles of meditation, so these studies were categorized as "various" styles of meditation.

Not only did the type of meditation studied vary, but there was also a range of imaging techniques used across the studies. Gray matter volume and gray matter concentration were two common methods to look at the quantity of gray matter in different brain regions. Gray matter contains a large number of neuronal cell bodies as well as blood vessels, unmyelinated axons and non-neuronal cells.

> **Remind me...are larger brain regions better?**
> Although it may seem better to have larger brain regions, neuroscientists still don't fully understand how brain size affects function. For example, a larger brain region could mean that a person has more neurons, more blood vessels or more support cells. Conversely, a smaller brain region could mean a person's brain is more efficient, as Einstein's brain was thought to be (Costandi, 2012).
>
> Studies do suggest that larger brain regions, in general, may be a good thing. Cognitive development is linked to larger brain regions whereas brain cell death, neurodegenerative diseases and cognitive decline are linked to shrinking brain regions (Smale *et al.*, 1995).

Another common method used in the studies reviewed was diffusion tensor imaging, which highlights white matter (axons) tracts in the brain. Other methods included measuring the cortical thickness and the cortical gyrification, which are other ways to measure gray matter (Figure 7.2). Unfortunately, when so many different techniques are used, the results can be hard to compare (Fox *et al.*, 2014). So, the researchers focused on the brain regions that stood out across all the studies.

The researchers found nine main brain regions that were significantly different in at least three or more of the studies reviewed. Six brain regions appeared to be related to meditation practice. These included the insula (interoception or sensing the internal state of the body), the **somatomotor cortices** (sensory regions involved in body awareness), the prefrontal cortex (executive function/attention), the cingulate cortex (emotion regulation), the hippocampus (memory) and the **corpus callosum** (hemisphere-to-hemisphere communication).

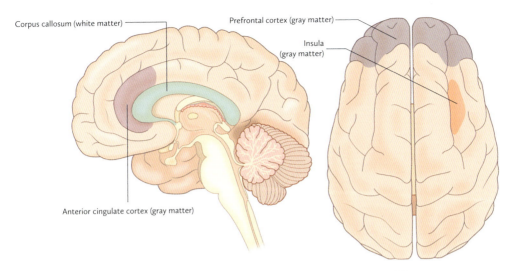

Figure 7.2 Brain structure differences in meditation practitioners.

The insula is consistently associated with meditation across the neuroimaging literature. Brain structure differences in the insula of meditators are also some of the most replicated findings, according to the authors of the study (Fox et al., 2014). The insula is associated with awareness and interoception, two key features of meditation. Awareness includes noticing the breath and heart rate, psychological states and self-awareness. The authors note that many of the studies that showed anatomical differences in the insula were studies where the meditators focused on body awareness, such as in Vipassana or insight meditation (Fox et al., 2014). These findings suggest that meditation may rely on the insula to sense the state of the body.

The somatomotor cortices are regions of the brain involved in processing tactile information, such as touch and pain. Since meditators appear to have more bodily awareness, they may also have a heightened sense of tactile inputs, like touch. Long-term meditators have a higher pain tolerance than non-meditators, and mindfulness meditation is used to help reduce chronic pain (Liu et al., 2012; Hilton et al., 2016). These brain structure differences could underlie the ability of meditators to reduce the feeling of pain through directed body awareness and acceptance (Fox et al., 2014).

The prefrontal cortex was reported as being structurally different than in the control group participants in three of the studies reviewed. These studies examined insight meditation, Tibetan Buddhist meditation and Brain Wave Vibration meditation, which are all quite different practices. For example, insight meditation is a form of mindfulness meditation, Tibetan Buddhist meditation involves mantras and visualizations, and Brain Wave Vibration meditation entails moving the head, neck and body with yoga-related exercises (Bowden, McLennan and Gruzelier, 2014). The prefrontal cortex has many diverse roles that involve decision making and processing emotions. It may also play a role in self-monitoring, which is a key feature of many types of meditation and could explain why it was structurally different in meditators in comparison with the control groups.

The cingulate cortex is commonly identified in meditation research. The cingulate cortex is involved in emotion regulation and, possibly, self-regulation. Since many types of meditation involve emotion regulation, this region might be anatomically different in people who regularly meditate.

Five of the reviewed studies showed brain structure differences in the hippocampus of meditators when compared with a control group. Beyond its role in memory, the hippocampus is also involved in emotional learning and stress. Repeated stress triggers inflammation, which bathes the hippocampus in cortisol. This process leads to cell death and reduces functioning of the hippocampus. Hippocampal dysfunction is linked to neurodegenerative diseases, such as Alzheimer's disease, as well as many psychiatric disorders, like anxiety and depression. Regular meditation practice could protect this region against stress, as meditation cultivates resilience and trains the mind to become less reactive to stress.

The corpus callosum, the bridge between the two hemispheres, also showed some brain structure differences in meditators. This information highway is made up of white matter tracts (neuronal axons) that send information back and forth to the two halves (hemispheres) of the brain. Meditators may have better connectivity between brain regions. The authors suggest increased gray matter (cell bodies) in some regions could mean the brain needs more white matter (axons) to carry those signals around the brain (Fox *et al*., 2014). Thus, meditators may have increased communication and synchronization across brain regions than those who do not meditate.

It is difficult to know whether meditation *causes* brain structure changes, or if differences in brain structure lead people to take up meditation in the first place (Fox *et al*., 2014). Regardless, many studies do suggest that certain brain regions are different in those who meditate. The causal nature of the relationship will need to be explored in future studies.

Main takeaways
- Meditation is often categorized into four main categories which include: 1) focused-attention meditation, 2) mantra recitation meditation, 3) loving-kindness meditation, and 4) open monitoring meditation.
- Practicing meditation may alter multiple brain structures. Some of the most common brain regions related to practicing meditation include the insula, the somatomotor cortices, the prefrontal cortex, the cingulate cortex, the hippocampus and the corpus callosum.

Does meditation experience matter?

Most studies about the neuroanatomy of meditation focus on differences in gray matter as well as cortical thickness. Another way to look at neuroanatomy is by examining the gyrification of the brain (Figure 7.3). **Gyrification** refers to the pattern and degree of cortical folding (Luders *et al*., 2012). In other words, it is a measure of the wrinkles in the brain's surface.

Neuroscientists believe gyrification is an indicator of the number of neurons in the brain. For example, more folding suggests more gray matter with more neurons. This theory is supported by the fact that some less intelligent primates, such as howler monkeys, have almost smooth brains, suggesting fewer neurons. In contrast, the human brain is riddled with folds and grooves.

In a study of 100 participants, scientists from the University of California, Los Angeles School of Medicine and the University of Jena in Germany examined the cortical gyrification between meditators and controls to see if there were any brain differences (Luders *et al*., 2012). Notably, they found that meditators had more gyrification in the insula than the control group. They also found that meditators with more experience had more gyrification of their insula than meditators with less experience (Figure 7.4). The findings suggest that meditation appears related to gyrification in this region, especially in more experienced meditators.

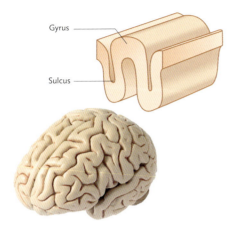

Figure 7.3 Gyrification of the brain.
Adapted from: Lobes of the brain, Queensland Brain Institute. From: https://qbi.uq.edu.au/brain/brain-anatomy/lobes-brain

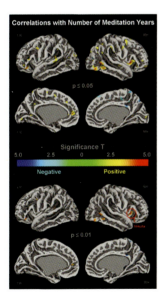

Figure 7.4 Cortical gyrification is related to the number of meditation years in the insula (labeled in red).
Source: Luders et al., 2012, originally published by Frontiers, CC BY 4.0. From: https://www.frontiersin.org/articles/10.3389/fnhum.2012.00034/full

This study was cross-sectional, meaning that it only examined the meditators' brains at one time point. Thus, it is impossible to determine if the increased gyrification of the insula is due to meditation practice or not. Instead, it could be that people with more gyrification in their insula are more likely to practice meditation in the first place (Luders et al., 2012). Although the results seem promising, more studies will need to be conducted to confirm these results.

To get a better idea of how long-term meditation affects brain structure, researchers from the University of Auckland in New Zealand conducted a review where they examined all of the neuroimaging studies that compared long-term meditators with controls (Luders and Kurth, 2019). Their analysis included 12 studies with participants who had an average of 10 years of meditation practice.

The review showed that long-term meditators had larger brain regions (more gray matter, cortical thickness, etc.) than the control groups in multiple brain areas. A few regions stood out in three or more studies as being significantly different than in the control group: the prefrontal cortex, insula and hippocampus. These three regions are often identified in meditation studies due to their role in executive function, interoception and memory, respectively.

Main takeaways
- **Gyrification** is the pattern and degree of cortical folding of the brain or how wrinkly the brain's surface appears. It is likely a measure of how many neurons there are in the brain.
- Experienced meditators show increased gyrification in their insula when compared with less experienced meditators and controls.
- Experienced meditators may also have larger brain regions than the control

participants. These areas include the prefrontal cortex, insula and hippocampus.

How does a brain region become larger?

Brain differences that can be observed using neuroimaging techniques require lots of changes on the cellular level. However, these cellular changes remain very poorly understood, especially in humans.

Scientists have proposed a few possibilities. In mouse models, one study found that larger volumes were correlated with more axons and axon reorganization, suggesting that brain region growth may be largely related to axons (white matter) instead of neuronal cell bodies (gray matter) (Fox et al., 2014).

Some researchers have suggested that new neurons might be created in these regions; however, this theory is likely incorrect. The process of creating new neurons in the brain is called neurogenesis, and multiple well-designed studies have suggested that neurogenesis is primarily restricted to the hippocampus (Kempermann, Song and Gage, 2015). Neurogenesis does not occur in regions such as the insula or the cingulate cortex.

One of the most limiting factors in understanding what causes brain volume changes or differences is that researchers cannot dissect the brain of human meditators. Thus, there is no direct way to see how meditation affects the brain on a microscopic level. Additionally, animal models are limited for studying practices like meditation because mice and rats cannot be taught to meditate. We may never fully understand the cellular changes that occur due to meditation, but advances in neuroimaging do help provide some insight into what might be occurring.

MEDITATION AFFECTS BRAIN FUNCTION

So far, we've looked at the structural differences, like brain size, density and gyrification, of the brains of meditators in comparison with control groups. Another way to examine the brain is to look at differences in how the brain functions during specific tasks, like meditation. To analyze brain function, the task must be completed inside a brain imaging machine, like an MRI scanner. MRIs are narrow and require the patient to lie flat and still. Thus, movement practices like yoga cannot be done inside an MRI scanner to look at brain function. However, one can easily meditate while researchers look at blood flow to different regions in the brain.

The same group of researchers from the University of British Columbia who conducted the review and meta-analysis of the neuroanatomy of meditation also examined the meditation studies related to brain function in a second review (Fox et al., 2016). For this project, the scientists included 78 studies with a total of 527 participants.

Across the studies reviewed, focused-attention meditation consistently activated the premotor cortex and the anterior cingulate cortex, which are associated with cognitive control and self-reflection, respectively. The scientists also note that, although not statistically significant, the dorsolateral prefrontal cortex and the insula were activated just below threshold levels (Fox et al., 2016). The dorsolateral prefrontal cortex is involved in the regulation of attention, which makes sense given that focused-attention meditation requires sustained attention. The insula is the region of the brain involved in the awareness of bodily sensations and interoception.

Mantra meditation was associated with activation in multiple brain regions involved in planning and the control of movement, including the dorsolateral prefrontal cortex, fusiform gyrus, cuneus and the precuneus. These regions may also be involved in reciting a mantra, either out loud or in one's head, the authors state (Fox et al., 2016). Interestingly, the insula was deactivated during mantra meditation, suggesting that awareness of the body is decreased during mantra meditation.

Open monitoring meditation showed brain activations in the insula as well as in multiple regions associated with voluntary movement, such as the inferior frontal gyrus, the pre-supplementary motor area, the supplementary motor area and the premotor cortex. The thalamus was shown to be deactivated during this type of meditation. The thalamus is a key relay station in the brain for processing sensory information. Thus, sensory processing could be dampened during open monitoring meditation.

Lastly, loving-kindness meditation showed activation in the insula and somatosensory areas of the brain. The insula is the region of the brain invoked in empathy, which is a key component of loving-kindness meditation, while the somatosensory cortex processes information about our senses. Loving-kindness meditation involves cultivating positive thoughts, such as joy and compassion, towards others and oneself. Loving-kindness meditation activates the same brain regions involved in these processes.

A few brain regions showed consistent activation across the four categories of meditation styles (Figure 7.5). The insula, which is involved in self-awareness and empathy, was implicated in all of the meditation styles. The insula had the most activation during the open monitoring meditation and the loving-kindness meditation. The insula showed less activity during the mantra meditation, which likely requires less of a focus on conscious awareness of the body since the practitioner is focusing on the mantra.

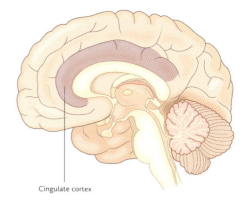

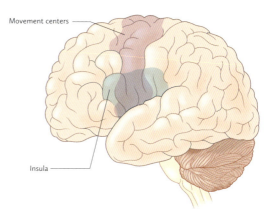

Figure 7.5 Summary of the activations and deactivations across all four categories of meditation. The three regions with consistent activation during all types of meditation were the insula, the movement centers and the cingulate cortex.

Many regions of the brain involved in movement showed activation during the various styles of meditation. This was an unexpected finding since the subjects were lying still during the neuroimaging. Recent research suggests that some movement areas of the brain may also play a role in cognition and attention, although more studies still need to be conducted (Fox et al., 2016).

The results also showed that the cingulate cortex plays a role in both focused-attention meditation and open monitoring meditation. The cingulate cortex is involved in the emotional response as well as attention and is likely involved in meditations that require regulation and monitoring.

> **Main takeaways**
> - **Focused-attention meditation** is associated with activation in the premotor cortex and the anterior cingulate cortex.
> - **Mantra meditation** is related to activation in brain regions involved in planning and the control of movement.
> - **Open monitoring meditation** showed brain activations in the insula as well as in multiple regions associated with voluntary movement.
> - **Loving-kindness meditation** showed more activity in the insula and somatosensory areas of the brain.
> - The insula and the cingulate cortex may play a role across all forms of meditation practices.

Brain networks involved in meditation

The brain largely functions in networks of brain regions, instead of single regions operating independently. One of the most frequently activated brain networks is the one used during periods of rest, called **resting-state networks**. These are active when the brain is not engaged in a specific activity or task.

Researchers from the University of Naples examined the effect of Vipassana meditation, a type of open monitoring mindfulness meditation, on resting-state brain networks (Lardone et al., 2018). The scientists were curious to see if meditation could alter the baseline way that a brain functions. The participants in the study included 26 regular Vipassana meditators, who had been practicing at least five days per week for at least a year, and 29 controls who had never meditated before.

They used a technique called magnetoencephalography (MEG), which is a noninvasive way to measure the magnetic fields produced by neurons' electrical currents. MEG is similar to electroencephalography (EEG); however, instead of measuring the magnetic fields of extracellular currents (currents outside the cells), MEG records the magnetic fields of intracellular currents (currents inside the cells) (Singh, 2014).

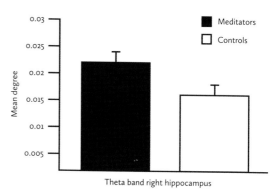

Figure 7.6 Meditators showed a higher degree in the theta band of the right hippocampus than the control group.

The researchers found that, when looking at brain waves from the whole brain, there were no real differences between the meditators and the control group. However, when they started to compare specific regions of the brain, they observed that the meditators showed a higher degree in the theta band of the right hippocampus than the control group (Figure 7.6).

The higher degree means that the hippocampus may be more connected to the rest of the resting network or more prominent in meditators than in the controls. The authors argue that this finding suggests that the hippocampus plays a key role in Vipassana meditation, which has been shown in other studies examining the brains of meditators (Lardone et al., 2018). Since the finding was only in the right hippocampus, the scientists speculate that this result could be because the right and left hippocampus function in slightly different ways or that they demonstrate different patterns of connectivity (Lardone et al., 2018).

THE DEFAULT MODE NETWORK

One type of resting-state network is called the **default mode network**. It includes parts of the prefrontal cortex, cingulate cortex, temporal lobe and hippocampus that are active when the brain is not engaged in a goal-oriented task. These regions have coordinated activity and tend to be less active during tasks that require cognitive effort and concentration. The default mode network is involved in self-related thinking and mind wandering (Garrison et al., 2015).

Practicing meditation can alter the default mode network. One study conducted by researchers from the Yale University School of Medicine found reduced default mode network activity across three types of meditation, including focused-attention, loving-kindness and open monitoring (called choiceless awareness by the authors) (Brewer et al., 2011).

The same group of scientists later replicated the study with a larger sample size, which included 20 experienced insight meditators and 26 controls to confirm their earlier results (Garrison et al., 2015). The experienced meditators reported an average of 10,000 hours of meditation practice over the past two years, and the control group had never meditated before.

Before going into the MRI brain scanner, the meditators were instructed to perform one of three styles of meditation, including focused-attention meditation, loving-kindness meditation and open monitoring meditation. Below are examples of the instructions as provided by the authors of the study (Garrison et al., 2015).

1. Focused-attention: "Please pay attention to the physical sensation of the breath wherever you feel it most strongly in the body. Follow the natural and spontaneous movement of the breath, not trying to change it in any way. Just pay attention to it. If you find that your attention has wandered to something else, gently but firmly bring it back to the physical sensation of the breath."
2. Loving-kindness: "Please think of a time when you genuinely wished someone well (pause). Using this feeling as a focus, silently wish all beings well, by repeating a few short phrases of your choosing over and over. For example: May all beings be happy, may all beings be healthy, may all beings be safe from harm."
3. Open monitoring: "Please pay attention to whatever comes into your awareness, whether it is a thought, emotion, or body sensation. Just follow it until something else comes into your awareness, not trying to hold onto it or change it in any way. When something else comes into your awareness, just pay attention to it until the next thing comes along."

The meditators were able to practice their instructed style of meditation before entering the brain scanner. The participants then entered the MRI scanner and performed two rounds of meditation, while the scientists examined which parts of their brains were receiving the most blood flow.

Overall, the experienced meditators reported less mind wandering than the control group during the meditation task. During meditation, two areas of the prefrontal cortex (the rectal gyrus and the orbitofrontal cortex) were observed to have increases in activity when compared with baseline. Meditators also showed less default mode network activity when compared with an active task and rest. These findings support the idea that meditators may have more control over their default mode network activity and can more easily turn it off when focusing on their meditation practice (Garrison et al., 2015).

Mantra meditation has been studied less than

other forms of meditation, but some scientists believe practicing this form of meditation may also alter default mode network functioning. Researchers from Linköping University in Sweden asked participants to take part in a two-week Kundalini yoga and mantra meditation to see how this practice affected the default mode network (Simon *et al.*, 2017). Each session started with yoga exercise and ended with 11 minutes of mantra meditation. The participants also performed finger-tapping to provide an attention-focused task for comparison.

The scientists found that the participants' default mode networks were more suppressed during the meditation than when performing the finger-tapping (Simon *et al.*, 2017). Thus, mantra meditation reduces mind wandering by decreasing the activity of the default mode network. Their findings are in line with other studies that found that focused-attention and open monitoring meditations also have a suppressive effect on the default mode network.

Considering these results, meditation may lessen self-related thinking and mind wandering by decreasing activity of the default mode network. An overly active default mode network is associated with neuropsychological conditions, such as depression and anxiety (Garrison *et al.*, 2015). Thus, this mechanism of reducing default mode network activity through meditation could be why meditation has been shown to be beneficial for people with these conditions.

> **Main takeaways**
> - **Resting-state networks** are brain regions that are active when the brain is not engaged in a specific task or activity. The hippocampus of meditators may function slightly differently during rest than in people who do not meditate.
> - The **default mode network** is active when the brain is not engaged in a goal-oriented task and includes coordinated regions such as the prefrontal cortex, cingulate cortex, temporal lobe and hippocampus.
> - Focused-attention, loving-kindness, open monitoring and mantra meditation styles reduce activity of the default mode network, which is thought to be neuroprotective.

Brain activity

Electroencephalography (EEG) is another common method for examining the brain. Unlike MRI, which is an indirect measure of blood flow, EEG detects the electrical activity of large groups of the brain's neurons. During an EEG, electrodes are placed on the scalp of an individual while they perform a task. EEGs can be a useful tool for understanding brain disorders, such as epilepsy, and are commonly used in research.

An EEG measures waves of signals of varying frequency, amplitude and shape. There are five main types of brain waves: gamma, beta, alpha, theta and delta waves (Figure 7.7).

Many meditation studies have examined the brain using EEG and found increased theta waves associated with the practice (Brandmeyer, Delorme and Wahbeh, 2019). Theta waves, which measure 4–8 Hz, are associated with relaxation and inward contemplation. Additionally, some studies have shown increases in alpha waves, which are associated with reduced symptoms of anxiety and an increase in feelings of calm. Other studies have shown increases in high-frequency gamma waves, which are associated with attention and concentration (Brandmeyer, Delorme and Wahbeh, 2019).

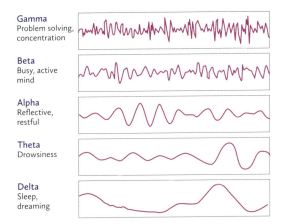

Figure 7.7 Characteristics of the five main types of brain waves.

Scientists from the University of Plymouth in the UK wanted to know if certain styles of meditation showed the same brain wave activity when compared with a control group (Braboszcz et al., 2017). They used EEG to examine the brain waves of practitioners of Vipassana, Himalayan Yoga and Isha Shoonya. Vipassana is a style of mindfulness meditation (sitting meditation), Himalayan Yoga is a meditation-based yoga style (movement with meditation), and Isha Shoonya is an open-awareness meditative style (meditation after movement) (Braboszcz et al., 2013).

The scientists found that every meditator showed higher gamma amplitudes (60–110 Hz) than the control group during meditation. Further, the more experienced meditators showed even higher gamma amplitudes than those with less experience. These findings align with another study which found more experienced Vipassana meditators, particularly those with more than 10 years of experience, had higher gamma wave power (Cahn, Delorme and Polich, 2009). The team also observed that Vipassana meditators showed higher alpha wave activity than all of the other groups during meditation (Braboszcz et al., 2017). These findings demonstrate how meditation can alter brain waves to create a state of calm and relaxation, especially in those with more meditation experience.

Main takeaways
- **Electroencephalography** (EEG) detects the electrical activity of large groups of neurons in the brain.
- There are five main types of brain waves: gamma, beta, alpha, theta and delta.
- Studies have shown increased theta, alpha and gamma waves with meditation practice. Theta waves are associated with relaxation and inward contemplation, while alpha waves are related to feeling calm, and gamma waves are linked with attention and concentration.
- Experienced meditators have higher alpha wave and gamma wave activity while meditating, suggesting they can become calmer and more focused during this practice than less experienced meditators.

REFERENCES

Bowden, D.E., McLennan, D., & Gruzelier, J., 2014. A randomised controlled trial of the effects of brain wave vibration training on mood and well-being. *Journal of Complementary and Integrative Medicine*, 11(3), pp.223–232.

Braboszcz, C., Cahn, B.R., Balakrishnan, B., Maturi, R.K., Grandchamp, R., & Delorme, A., 2013. Plasticity of visual attention in Isha Yoga meditation practitioners before and after a 3-month retreat. *Frontiers in Psychology*, 4.

Braboszcz, C., Cahn, B.R., Levy, J., Fernandez, M., & Delorme, A., 2017. Increased gamma brainwave amplitude compared to control in three different meditation traditions. *PLoS ONE*, 12(1), e0170647.

Brandmeyer, T., Delorme, A., & Wahbeh, H., 2019. The neuroscience of meditation: classification, phenomenology, correlates, and mechanisms. *Progress in Brain Research*, 244, pp.1-29.

Brewer, J.A., Worhunsky, P.D., Gray, J.R., Tang, Y., Weber, J., & Kober, H., 2011. Meditation experience is associated with differences in default mode network activity and connectivity. *Proceedings of the National Academy of Sciences*, 108(50), pp.20254-20259.

Cahn, B.R., Delorme, A., & Polich, J., 2009. Occipital gamma activation during Vipassana meditation. *Cognitive Processing*, 11(1), pp.39-56.

Carlson, L.E., & Garland, S.N., 2005. Impact of mindfulness-based stress reduction (MBSR) on sleep, mood, stress and fatigue symptoms in cancer outpatients. *International Journal of Behavioral Medicine*, 12(4), pp.278-285.

Chiesa, A., 2010. Vipassana meditation: systematic review of current evidence. *The Journal of Alternative and Complementary Medicine*, 16(1), pp.37-46.

Costandi, M., 2012. Snapshots explore Einstein's unusual brain. *Nature*. https://doi.org/10.1038/nature.2012.11836

Emavardhana, T., & Tori, C.D., 1997. Changes in self-concept, ego defense mechanisms, and religiosity following seven-day Vipassana meditation retreats. *Journal for the Scientific Study of Religion*, 36(2), p.194.

Fox, K.C.R., Nijeboer, S., Dixon, M.L., Floman, J.L., et al., 2014. Is meditation associated with altered brain structure? A systematic review and meta-analysis of morphometric neuroimaging in meditation practitioners. *Neuroscience & Biobehavioral Reviews*, 43, pp.48-73.

Fox, K.C.R., Dixon, M.L., Nijeboer, S., Girn, M., et al., 2016. Functional neuroanatomy of meditation: a review and meta-analysis of 78 functional neuroimaging investigations. *Neuroscience & Biobehavioral Reviews*, 65, pp.208-228.

Garrison, K.A., Zeffiro, T.A., Scheinost, D., Constable, R.T., & Brewer, J.A., 2015. Meditation leads to reduced default mode network activity beyond an active task. *Cognitive, Affective, & Behavioral Neuroscience*, 15(3), pp.712-720.

Goldin, P.R., & Gross, J.J., 2010. Effects of mindfulness-based stress reduction (MBSR) on emotion regulation in social anxiety disorder. *Emotion*, 10(1), pp.83-91.

Harrington, A., & Dunne, J.D., 2015. When mindfulness is therapy: ethical qualms, historical perspectives. *American Psychologist*, 70(7), pp.621-631.

Hilton, L., Hempel, S., Ewing, B.A., Apaydin, E., et al., 2016. Mindfulness meditation for chronic pain: systematic review and meta-analysis. *Annals of Behavioral Medicine*, 51(2), pp.199-213.

Kempermann, G., Song, H., & Gage, F.H., 2015. Neurogenesis in the adult hippocampus. *Cold Spring Harbor Perspectives in Biology*, 7(9), a018812.

Lardone, A., Liparoti, M., Sorrentino, P., Rucco, R., Jacini, F., Polverino, A., et al., 2018. Mindfulness meditation is related to long-lasting changes in hippocampal functional topology during resting state: a magnetoencephalography study. *Neural Plasticity*, 2018, pp.1-9.

Lazar, S.W., Kerr, C.E., Wasserman, R.H., Gray, J.R., Greve, D.N., Treadway, M.T., et al., 2005. Meditation experience is associated with increased cortical thickness. *NeuroReport*, 16(17), pp.1893-1897.

Liu, X., Wang, S., Chang, S., Chen, W., & Si, M., 2012. Effect of brief mindfulness intervention on tolerance and distress of pain induced by cold-pressor task. *Stress and Health*, 29(3), pp.199-204.

Luders, E., Kurth, F., Mayer, E.A., Toga, A.W., Narr, K.L., & Gaser, C., 2012. The unique brain anatomy of meditation practitioners: alterations in cortical gyrification. *Frontiers in Human Neuroscience*, 6, p.34.

Luders, E., & Kurth, F., 2019. The neuroanatomy of long-term meditators. *Current Opinion in Psychology*, 28, pp.172-178.

Moran, S., 2018. The science behind finding your mantra – and how to practice it daily. *Yoga Journal*. Available at: https://www.yogajournal.com/yoga-101/mantras-101-the-science-behind-finding-your-mantra-and-how-to-practice-it/

Owens, L.R., 2021. How to practice Shamatha meditation. *Lion's Roar*. Available at: https://www.lionsroar.com/how-to-practice-shamatha/

Pagnoni, G., & Cekic, M., 2007. Age effects on gray matter volume and attentional performance in Zen meditation. *Neurobiology of Aging*, 28(10), pp.1623-1627.

Rosenzweig, S., Greeson, J.M., Reibel, D.K., Green, J.S., Jasser, S.A., & Beasley, D., 2010. Mindfulness-based stress reduction for chronic pain conditions: variation in treatment outcomes and role of home meditation practice. *Journal of Psychosomatic Research*, 68(1), pp.29-36.

Simon, R., Pihlsgård, J., Berglind, U., Söderfeldt, B., & Engström, M., 2017. Mantra meditation suppression of default mode beyond an active task: a pilot study. *Journal of Cognitive Enhancement*, 1(2), pp.219-227.

Singh, S.P., 2014. Magnetoencephalography: basic principles. *Annals of Indian Academy of Neurology*, 17(5), p.107.

Smale, G., Nichols, N.R., Brady, D.R., Finch, C.E., & Horton Jr., W.E., 1995. Evidence for apoptotic cell death in Alzheimer's disease. *Experimental Neurology*, 133(2), pp.225-230.

CHAPTER 8

Stress, Trauma and Resilience

Many people begin a yoga or meditation practice to control or reduce their levels of stress (Figure 8.1). In this chapter, we will explore how stress affects the brain and body to better target it with effective contemplative practices. We will also examine what happens when stress becomes trauma and how to cultivate resilience with our practices.

STRESS

Stress is a state of mental, emotional or physical strain resulting from adverse or demanding circumstances. Although the word "stress" often has a negative connotation, stress in small doses, called acute stress, can be beneficial. For example, if you're a yoga teacher trying to come up with a new routine for class, a little stress might help you stay focused and work harder to finish your prep.

While some stress is normal, prolonged stress can be debilitating. Scientists believe the brain is designed to think about the future to make decisions that allow us to survive. However, if these worries persist too long or too intensely, we can develop mental health conditions, like anxiety and depression. Chronic stress can deplete the body of its resources without replenishment.

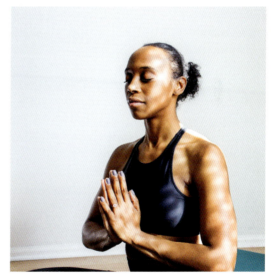

Figure 8.1 Meditation and yoga can help to reduce stress.
Source: Madison Lavern on Unsplash.

111

HOW THE NERVOUS SYSTEM RESPONDS TO STRESS

Stress can be triggered by a real threat, such as encountering a grizzly bear, or a perceived threat, like thinking that a grizzly bear *might* be lurking nearby. The body processes both real and perceived threats in a similar manner, and it releases a cascade of stress hormones to initiate the stress response.

The autonomic nervous system governs our stress response, which includes the sympathetic and parasympathetic nervous systems. These systems work together to maintain a state of equilibrium in the body called homeostasis.

When the brain senses a real or perceived danger, the sympathetic nervous system becomes activated as part of the "fight, flight or freeze" response. The body prepares to either escape from the danger, fight off the danger, or freeze to avoid being seen or to play dead. Once the sympathetic nervous system is activated, the heart rate increases, muscles tense, breathing quickens, sweat appears, and blood and nutrients are shunted away from resting processes, such as digestion, towards systems involved in preparing for active response, such as the skeletal muscles. During this time, the parasympathetic nervous system is essentially on standby until the danger is gone. After the danger has ended, the sympathetic nervous system becomes less active, and the parasympathetic nervous system revs up, bringing the body back into equilibrium.

This involuntary reaction is characteristic of acute stress. During long-term or chronic stress, the sympathetic nervous system stays perpetually active, causing physical stress on the body over time. Some of the symptoms of chronic stress include muscle pains, exhaustion, insomnia, headaches, dizziness, digestive problems and a weakened immune system. Mental health conditions, such as anxiety and depression, and neurodegenerative disorders, like Alzheimer's disease and Parkinson's disease, are thought to also be related to chronic stress (Liu, Wang and Jiang, 2017).

The brain's stress system

Neuroscientists believe that stress alters multiple neurotransmitters, hormones and chemicals in the brain starting in the amygdala. During stress, the amygdala may become more active, triggering the sympathetic nervous system and a major stress pathway called the **hypothalamic-pituitary-adrenal (HPA) axis** (Liu, Wang and Jiang, 2017). The HPA axis describes the interaction between the hypothalamus, the pituitary gland (located under the hypothalamus) and the adrenal glands (located on top of both kidneys), which all work together to help regulate the body's stress response by releasing a cascade of hormones.

When the brain senses stress, the hypothalamus releases a hormone called corticotropin-releasing hormone (CRH) that signals to the pituitary gland that the stress system needs to be activated. The pituitary gland responds by releasing the hormone adrenocorticotrophic hormone (ACTH) into the bloodstream.

ACTH travels to the adrenal glands telling them to get to work, and the adrenals respond by releasing stress hormones, including epinephrine, norepinephrine and cortisol into the bloodstream (Figure 8.2). These hormones travel quickly around the body. Receptors for the stress hormones are located on most cells and can quickly alter the heart rate, blood pressure and other bodily systems involved in the stress response.

Chronic stress can lead to elevated levels of stress hormones that persist over time. High levels of cortisol can damage cells in certain regions of the brain, such as the hippocampus. Too much cortisol in the hippocampus can cause structural changes and even cell death. These changes can have long-lasting effects and can alter memory, cognition and even future responses to stress (Lupien *et al.*, 2009).

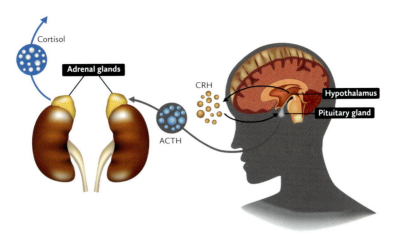

Figure 8.2 The hypothalamic-pituitary-adrenal (HPA) axis.

The sympathetic nervous system in action

An overactive sympathetic nervous system is not a good thing, but a normally functioning sympathetic nervous system is necessary for rigorous exercise. Intense physical exercise requires increased heart rate, and the blood vessels expand and contract to bring nutrients and oxygen to the muscles (Hearon and Dinenno, 2015). This response would not be possible without some level of activation of the sympathetic nervous system.

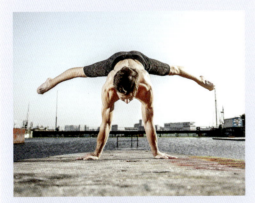

Figure 8.3 Intense exercise, which can include some yoga postures, activates the sympathetic nervous system.
Source: Patrick Kool on Unsplash.

The parasympathetic nervous system

Slower, more intentional movement practices and meditation target the parasympathetic nervous system, which allows the body to release tension and begin the process of restoration and nourishment.

The parasympathetic nervous system is the "rest and digest" system. Activation of this nervous system can stimulate muscles in the digestive tract to process food and slow the heart rate. The vagus nerve connects the parasympathetic nervous system to numerous organs throughout the body. The word *vagus* means "wandering" in Latin because it connects to so many different structures.

Meditation is a common method for activating the parasympathetic nervous system and reducing stress. A large review of the literature conducted by researchers from Johns Hopkins University, including 47 studies with 3,515 total participants, found that meditation may offer a plethora of stress-reducing health benefits (Goyal et al., 2014). The evidence showed that meditation programs were effective at reducing anxiety, depression, pain and stress levels. Meditation also improved overall mental health across the studies. However, it was unclear if meditation was more effective than other treatment options, such as exercise, medication or behavioral therapies. It is likely that all four approaches provide some level of benefit for reducing stress.

> **Main takeaways**
> - **Stress** is a state of mental, emotional or physical strain resulting from adverse or demanding circumstances.
> - While acute stress can be beneficial, chronic stress can deplete the body of its resources over time and lead to mental health conditions, like anxiety or depression.
> - The sympathetic nervous system is triggered when the brain senses a real or perceived threat.
> - The **hypothalamic-pituitary-adrenal (HPA) axis** is a stress pathway that becomes activated when the sympathetic nervous system is triggered. The HPA axis produces stress hormones, such as cortisol, that can damage the brain when released on a sustained basis.
> - Practicing meditation may offer a plethora of health benefits, such as reducing anxiety, depression, pain and stress.

CHRONIC STRESS AND INFLAMMATION

During chronic stress, the sympathetic nervous system and the HPA axis are repeatedly triggered to release more and more stress hormones. These hormones interfere with the body's homeostasis and can cause damage over time. It's like a leaky faucet that continues to trickle water into a sink. Cortisol levels can drastically rise and stay high for too long, leading to problems such as high blood pressure, increased blood glucose, immune suppression, depression and neuron death, especially in the hippocampus (Venkatesh et al., 2020). Sustained increases in epinephrine and norepinephrine can cause higher blood cholesterol and free fatty acid levels as well as suppress the immune system.

Sustained stress can also lead to **chronic inflammation**. Normally, inflammation is part of the immune response to fight offending agents like bacteria and viruses as well as start the healing process. However, during chronic inflammation the body releases inflammatory cells even when it is not being attacked or actively damaged. Chronic inflammation is a key component of chronic illness and stress-related diseases (Liu, Wang and Jiang, 2017).

Despite the strong association, there is still a lot to learn about the pathways connecting stress and inflammation. Scientists know stress can activate the inflammatory response in the brain as well as in the body (Liu, Wang and Jiang, 2017). One of the main neurotransmitters involved in this connection is norepinephrine, which is a key player in the sympathetic nervous system. Some research has shown that norepinephrine can increase the release of factors that promote inflammation (Gosain et al., 2006).

> **Common biomarkers of stress and inflammation**
> A **biomarker** is a measurable substance that is indicative of a biological state, such as stress or inflammation. Researchers use biomarkers to examine anything from the immune system to depression and Alzheimer's disease. For example, hemoglobin A1C is a commonly used biomarker for diabetes. These are some of the common biomarkers of stress and inflammation used in yoga research studies:

- Tumor necrosis factor alpha (TNF-α): a protein produced during inflammation that aids in resistance to infection and cancer. It can also produce signals that lead to cell death (Idriss and Naismith, 2000).
- Interleukin-6 (IL-6): a protein produced in response to infections and tissue damage. It is also involved in the inflammatory and immune response (Tanaka, Narazaki and Kishimoto, 2014).
- Interleukin-1β (IL-1β): a protein that is a key mediator of the inflammatory response and resistance to pathogens (Lopez-Castejon and Brough, 2011).
- C-reactive protein (CRP): a protein that is involved in the inflammatory and immune response. It is related to many inflammatory diseases, such as Alzheimer's disease and cardiovascular disease (Luan and Yao, 2018).

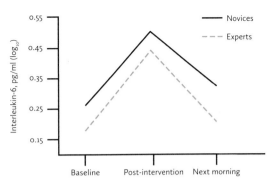

Figure 8.4 Expert yoga practitioners showed lower levels of the stress/inflammation biomarker interleukin-6 at baseline, after the yoga session (post-intervention), and the next morning, than the novice yoga practitioners.

Yoga can reduce both stress and inflammation. Researchers from Ohio State University College of Medicine examined the effect of yoga on hormone and inflammatory responses between novice and expert Hatha yoga practitioners to learn more about this connection (Kiecolt-Glaser et al., 2010). They found that, overall, the yoga sessions boosted participants' feeling of positivity. When the scientists compared the novice practitioners with the expert practitioners, the novices had 41 percent higher levels of a stress biomarker called interleukin-6 than the experts. The authors note that the differences in stress hormone levels could be explained by the years of practice (Figure 8.4). Expert practitioners may be able to better regulate their stress response, thereby reducing their inflammatory response, than the novice practitioners.

The same group of scientists conducted a rigorous randomized control trial which included 200 breast cancer survivors a few years later (Kiecolt-Glaser et al., 2014). They examined the effect of Hatha yoga on markers of inflammation (interleukin-6, tumor necrosis factor alpha and interleukin-1β) along with reported levels of fatigue, vitality and depression.

Participants were assigned to either the yoga condition (three months of 90-minute Hatha yoga twice a week) or a control condition. The scientists found that after three months of yoga, the participants had lower measures of inflammation (interleukin-6 and interleukin-1β, but not tumor necrosis factor alpha) and reported less fatigue than the control group. The results suggest that regularly practicing yoga can promote health by reducing multiple measures of inflammation. It is unclear why some measures of inflammation were reduced, while others were not.

In another study, scientists from the University of Nebraska Medical Center conducted a review of the literature to examine the impact of different styles of yoga on markers of inflammation (Djalilova et al., 2018). They included 15 studies in their review and found that most studies showed the yoga intervention decreased interleukin-6, C-reactive protein and tumor necrosis factor alpha. Additionally, the analysis showed that higher "doses" of yoga (>1,000 minutes of yoga practice per study) resulted in larger decreases in inflammation from baseline to post-yoga intervention. Overall, the results suggest that yoga can be a successful intervention for reducing inflammation.

Meditation is also an effective means of decreasing stress to reduce inflammation on a cellular level. Scientists from Harvard University and Massachusetts General Hospital examined how meditation affects the body's metabolism and inflammatory pathways (Bhasin et al., 2013). They found that meditating, even just one time, had the ability to diminish the effects of genes involved with the inflammatory and stress responses while promoting the activation of genes associated with metabolism and DNA longevity.

Generating compassion for others, such as during a loving-kindness meditation, can reduce markers of stress and inflammation, like cortisol (Buchanan et al., 2012). Scientists from Emory University and the University of Arizona examined how compassion training was associated with a marker of inflammation called C-reactive protein (Pace et al., 2013). In the study, 71 adolescents in the Georgia foster care system were randomly assigned to either six weeks of compassion training or a control group. Saliva samples were collected from the participants before and after the training to measure the levels of C-reactive protein. Although the groups didn't differ in their levels of C-reactive protein, within the compassion group, the number of sessions was related to reduced levels of the protein. Thus, more compassion training led to fewer inflammatory measures (Pace et al., 2013).

Mindfulness-based stress reduction can improve mood and psychological well-being. As these factors are related to immune system functioning, scientists from the Fox Chase Cancer Center in Pennsylvania set out to examine if mindfulness-based stress reduction could positively impact immune functioning (Fang et al., 2010). Twenty-four participants underwent a two-month mindfulness-based stress reduction course. Each class was 2.5 hours in length and participants were asked to practice 20–30 minutes of meditation at home most days of the week. Participants were tested at baseline and within two weeks after the conclusion of the mindfulness-based stress reduction course. Overall, participants reported significant improvements in their levels of anxiety, which was associated with a reduction in C-reactive protein. Individuals who reported improvement in their overall mental health showed increased natural killer cell cytolytic activity, a measure of immune activity.

Main takeaways
- Chronic stress can lead to health issues such as high blood pressure and the death of neurons in the brain.
- During **chronic inflammation**, the body releases inflammatory cells over an extended period of time.
- A **biomarker** is a measurable substance that is indicative of a biological state, such as stress or inflammation.
- Practicing yoga and meditation may reduce levels of inflammation in the body.

STRESS AND THE IMMUNE SYSTEM

Stress and the immune system are intricately intertwined. Mild, short-term stress can enhance the immune system, whereas intense or long-term stress can suppress it. Stress produces hormones that induce the inflammatory response, which suppresses the immune system. But when we talk about stress, it's not just physical stress that can affect the immune system, but also psychological stress. In fact, psychological stress is a major contributor to many inflammatory conditions (Rosenkranz et al., 2013).

Yoga and meditation can reduce psychological stress and, therefore, reduce the inflammatory response to improve immune system functioning. In a recent review of 15 randomized control trials examining the effects of yoga on the immune system, scientists found that yoga may downregulate pro-inflammatory markers, such as interleukin-1β (Falkenberg, Eising and Peters, 2018). Thus, yoga could be an effective tool for decreasing inflammation and improving the immune response. This finding is especially relevant for individuals with diseases that have an immune or inflammatory component, such as rheumatoid arthritis or Crohn's disease.

Mindfulness meditation may be superior to other forms of stress reduction. Scientists from the Waisman Laboratory for Brain Imaging & Behavior and Center for Investigating Healthy Minds at the University of Wisconsin-Madison sought to test the effectiveness of a mindfulness-based stress reduction (MBSR) intervention on stress and inflammation in comparison with a health promotion intervention called the Health Enhancement Program (Rosenkranz et al., 2013). The Health Enhancement Program is an active condition designed to be a control for MBSR-based studies, and it is identical to MBSR except without the mindfulness component.

Participants were assigned to either the MBSR group or the Health Enhancement Program group and completed their assigned two-month course. Psychological stress was induced using the Trier Social Stress Test, which is a trial where participants must deliver a speech and perform mental arithmetic in front of an audience (Kirschbaum, Pirke and Hellhammer, 1993), and inflammation was induced by applying capsaicin cream to the skin of the forearm. Capsaicin cream is made with the extract of hot peppers and can cause a warm, burning sensation.

The researchers measured levels of stress and inflammation before and after the trainings. Both groups showed increased levels of cortisol during the stress test and reductions in psychological and physical feelings of stress after the interventions. Although both groups showed similar levels of stress hormones, the MBSR group had less of an inflammatory response after the stress test than the Health Enhancement Program group. The authors note that the findings suggest that meditation could be beneficial for those with inflammatory conditions, and meditation could be even more effective at reducing inflammation than other health promoting interventions (Rosenkranz et al., 2013).

Another correlate of health and immune function used in research is the enzyme telomerase, a measure of cellular health (Epel et al., 2004). Telomerase acts to keep telomeres, the endcaps on chromosomes, from unraveling and stay long. Higher telomerase activity is associated with markers of better immune functioning, and longer telomeres are directly related to health and longevity (Wolkowitz et al., 2011).

Scientists from the University of New England in Australia conducted a review of studies involving mindfulness meditation and telomerase (Schutte and Malouff, 2014). The researchers found that across the four randomized control trials, which included 190 total participants, mindfulness meditation was associated with increased telomerase activity. The pooled results suggest that meditation can positively influence markers of cellular health and immune functioning (Schutte and Malouff, 2014).

> **Main takeaways**
> - Mild, short-term stress can enhance the immune system, whereas intense or long-term stress can suppress it.
> - Both physical and psychological stress can contribute to inflammation and suppression of the immune system.
> - Yoga and meditation can reduce markers of inflammation and improve immune system functioning. Meditation may be more effective than other health promoting programs and can alter the body's response to stress.
> - Meditation may benefit cellular health by increasing the activity of the enzyme telomerase.

THE TRAUMA-AFFECTED BRAIN

Although experiencing stress from time to time is healthy, intense stress can lead to detrimental effects on the brain. In the research literature, it can be unclear what the difference is between stressful and traumatic experiences. Scientists recently proposed that while stressful experiences can lead to resilience, traumatic experiences often lead to the development of psychopathologies, like anxiety and depression (Richter-Levin and Sandi, 2021). Traumatic experiences can be due to abuse, neglect and violence, among other things, and may physically affect the brain. Certain brain regions can shrink, while other regions grow, and circuits become rewired in response to traumatic events.

Trauma can also alter how the brain responds to stress. With too much stress, the amygdala can become overactive, telling the body that it is constantly in danger. Once the amygdala becomes hyperactive, it can be more easily triggered by lower levels of stress. This can lead to exaggerated responses when faced with even a mild stressor.

The decision center, the prefrontal cortex, can also shut down during intense stress, leading to issues with decision making, concentration and learning. Intense stress can cause changes in the anterior cingulate cortex, a region that helps regulate emotions. Over time, it can become more and more difficult to manage emotions during a stressful moment than it was prior to the intense stress exposure. For example, if someone is scared, they might remain scared long after the trigger is removed.

These long-term consequences of trauma can be especially detrimental for children. Children who experience trauma early in life may be more susceptible to mental health disorders, such as anxiety, post-traumatic stress disorder and depression.

WHAT DOESN'T KILL YOU MAKES YOU STRONGER: CULTIVATING RESILIENCE

Resilience is the ability to recover or "bounce back" after experiencing stress. Like learning a skill, resilience can be cultivated and improved with practice. Contemplative practices, such as yoga and meditation, can alter how one experiences stress by increasing resilience.

For example, the coronavirus pandemic brought the world to a standstill in 2020. City streets became empty, highways were deserted, and industrialized nations went into lockdown. The isolation of extended periods of quarantine and lockdown in combination with the fear of becoming ill with COVID-19 tested people's mental health.

Women often took more of the burden as they now had to juggle working from home with childcare and education, since many daycares and schools were closed. Subsequently, women were at higher risk than men of developing symptoms of stress, anxiety and depression (Matiz et al., 2020).

Many people sought mind–body practices that they could practice in their own home to preserve their mental health. In Italy, researchers studied the effect of a two-month mindfulness-oriented meditation on the mental health of 66 female teachers during the coronavirus pandemic (Matiz et al., 2020). The scientists did not intentionally set out to study the effects of mindfulness during the coronavirus pandemic, but the timing of the study led to some important conclusions about the benefits of meditation during intense psychological distress.

Based on their personality profiles, the teachers were divided into high-resilience and low-resilience groups. The groups took self-report assessments one month before and one month after the start of the coronavirus outbreak. Both groups showed improvements in anxiety, depression, empathy, emotional exhaustion, well-being and mindfulness levels after the mindfulness-oriented meditation training. Improvements in symptoms of depression and well-being were higher in the low-resilience group than in the high-resilience group. The findings suggest that mindfulness meditation can significantly improve many aspects of mental health, even in vulnerable populations, such as in people with less resilience (Matiz et al., 2020).

Mindful meditation for resilience
Come to a comfortable position, resting the hands wherever they're comfortable. Start to notice the body, the weight of the body. Let yourself become more curious about the physical body. Notice any parts of the body that might have tension. Breathe into the tension, allowing it to gently float away. And now bring your attention to the breath. Where do you feel the breath in your body? Feel the air as it comes in through the nose and makes its way down into the lungs. Notice that same air as it travels back up and out the nose. Follow this natural flow of the breath. Focus on the sensations of the breath. Find the point where one breath ends, and the next breath begins. If your mind begins to wander, acknowledge the thought, and come back to the breath. If the mind wanders again, it's OK. Be kind to yourself. This is normal. Bring the focus back to the breath and allow it to guide you into a deeper state of calm. Stay here for a moment. Soak in the full moment. Be present. Slowly, with care, start to come back to the breath. Allow the breath to resemble waves as it comes in and out of the body. Ride the waves as you come back to the world around you. Start to wiggle the fingers and toes as you sense touch. Open the eyes if they were closed, and bathe in this new, relaxed self.

> **Main takeaways**
> - Traumatic experiences can lead to the development of pathologies, like anxiety and depression.
> - The amygdala and prefrontal cortex can be altered with exposure to traumatic stress, leading to changes in brain structure and function.
> - **Resilience** is the ability to recover or "bounce back" after experiencing stress.
> - Meditation can significantly improve many aspects of mental health, even in vulnerable populations, such as in people with less resilience.

ANXIETY

Anxiety disorders are one of the most common mental health conditions in the United States, affecting nearly one in five adults with women being twice as likely to be affected than men, according to the Anxiety and Depression Association of America (ADAA). Symptoms of **anxiety** include persistent and excessive worrying, irrational fear and panic attacks. Anxiety can be successfully treated through medication, cognitive behavioral therapy and other means, yet only 43 percent of people receive any sort of treatment (ADAA, 2022).

What causes anxiety?

Despite the prevalence of anxiety disorders in the United States, scientists are still trying to understand the mechanisms involved in the condition. Anxiety disorders are characterized by a variety of disruptions in neuroendocrine systems, neurotransmitters and neuroanatomy (Martin *et al.*, 2009). They are thought to stem from an imbalance in the emotional centers of the brain and likely involve the amygdala.

The emotional centers of the brain are collectively known as the limbic system. Two of these brain regions, the insula and the cingulate cortex, are involved in integrating sensory and mood information as well as cognitive aspects of pain and internal awareness, also known as interoception. The memory center, the hippocampus, can reduce the activity of the hypothalamic-pituitary (HPA) axis, and the amygdala is involved in initiating the fear response and the retrieval of fear-related memories. Imaging studies have shown that individuals with anxiety tend to have larger amygdalas than those without anxiety (Martin *et al.*, 2009). These brain regions act together to form the limbic system, which processes the emotional response. When this system gets disrupted, the mood can become destabilized.

Neurotransmitters are the means of communication within and between brain regions. Scientists believe that over-communication or increased neurotransmitter activity can result in an anxiety disorder. The increased activity could be due to too much excitatory neurotransmission by glutamate, or a lack of inhibition by γ-amino-butyric-acid (GABA).

The neurotransmitters serotonin, norepinephrine and dopamine are also implicated in mood disorders. Scientists believe serotonin plays a role in mood disorders because serotonin reuptake inhibitors (SSRIs), which increase the levels of serotonin at the synapse (the location of communication between neurons), help reduce symptoms of anxiety and depression in many people.

Genetic and environmental factors, such as diet and exercise, can also play a role in susceptibility to developing anxiety. The same genes may be involved in multiple types of mood disorders, especially those that affect the HPA axis stress pathway. Environmental factors can directly affect gene expression to effectively turn genes on or off, resulting in a cascade of reactions leading to both physical and mental health conditions.

Yoga for anxiety

Yoga appears to be effective in reducing symptoms of anxiety in children, adolescents and young adults, but it may be less effective in adult populations. A review of yoga interventions for adolescents and children found that nearly all 16 studies analyzed showed reduced levels of anxiety after a yoga intervention (Weaver and Darragh, 2015). In an experimental study, researchers also found that that a six-week yoga and meditation intervention reduced stress and anxiety among college students (Lemay, Hoolahan and Buchanan, 2019). However, their study only consisted of 17 students, and there was no control group.

Although it seems logical that yoga would help to improve symptoms of anxiety, many studies have found conflicting results, especially in adult populations. A review of eight randomized control trials with a total of 319 participants showed that yoga did not appear to help those with anxiety diagnosed using the *Diagnostic and Statistical Manual* ("DSM," the standard book used by clinicians and psychiatrists in the United States for diagnosis) but did offer benefit to individuals without a formal diagnosis and those diagnosed by other methods (Cramer et al., 2018). Thus, yoga may be an effective intervention for those with high levels of subjective anxiety, but the evidence was less promising for those with formally diagnosed anxiety.

Another systematic review of 18 studies examined how Hatha yoga helped decrease severity of acute, chronic and/or treatment-resistant mood and anxiety disorders (Vollbehr et al., 2018). Fourteen of the studies were of patients with acute disorders, while four were of chronic disorders. The scientists found that Hatha yoga had no significant effect in decreasing symptoms of anxiety or depression when compared with the control groups. The authors acknowledge that most of the studies included in the review were low quality; therefore, more studies are needed to confirm or deny these results.

Meditation for anxiety

Mindfulness meditation is commonly recommended by therapists to help reduce symptoms of anxiety. And, unlike yoga, research does generally support that meditation can be a beneficial treatment aid. In 2013, researchers from Massachusetts General Hospital conducted the first randomized control trial comparing mindfulness-based stress reduction with an active control for generalized anxiety disorder (Hoge et al., 2013). Ninety-three participants with anxiety were assigned to either the eight-week meditation group or stress management education. Both interventions significantly reduced levels of anxiety; however, the meditation group showed a larger reduction in anxiety and distress ratings and a greater increase in positive self-statements than the control group. This was the first rigorous study to show how meditation can positively impact individuals with anxiety.

A review of the literature conducted in 2018 by scientists from the University of Heidelberg in Germany found that mindfulness-based interventions had a small to moderate effect on reducing symptoms of anxiety and depression, even without being a part of a larger therapeutic framework (Blanck et al., 2018). Their review consisted of 18 studies with a total of 1,150 participants. This review was the first meta-analysis to show that mindfulness-based interventions could benefit those with anxiety and depression, even if the intervention was not a part of therapy.

Most recently, researchers from Georgetown University and Harvard Medical School conducted a clinical trial, comparing participants who participated in an eight-week mindfulness meditation course with subjects who took escitalopram (the generic form of Lexapro), an anti-anxiety medication (Hoge et al., 2022). The study included 276 people diagnosed with untreated anxiety disorders. Half of them were assigned to the eight-week meditation course, while the other half started taking the anti-anxiety medication.

The results showed that both groups were able to reduce symptoms of anxiety by 20 percent. In other words, meditation worked as well as taking the medication for managing anxiety. The authors note that meditation could be a useful treatment strategy for those who do not wish to take medication or as a complementary treatment for those already taking medication (Hoge et al., 2022). Meditation could also be used as a first-line treatment, prior to starting medication. Thus, meditation may be an effective treatment option for those experiencing anxiety.

> **Main takeaways**
> - **Anxiety** is characterized by persistent and excessive worrying, irrational fear and panic attacks.
> - Yoga appears to be effective in reducing symptoms of anxiety in children, adolescents and young adults, but it may be less effective in adults.
> - Meditation has been shown across multiple studies to alleviate anxiety.

POST-TRAUMATIC STRESS DISORDER

Post-traumatic stress disorder (PTSD) is a trauma- or stress-related disorder that affects roughly 3.5 percent of the US population. It is a condition of persistent mental and emotional stress that can involve sleep disturbances and vivid recall of a stressful experience. PTSD can cause impairment of an individual's social interactions, capacity to work and daily functioning.

What causes PTSD?

The brain basis of PTSD is currently being studied by scientists, but they do know that the amygdala plays a key role in the fear learning aspect of PTSD (Martin et al., 2009). In PTSD, the amygdala is often over reactive and hypersensitive; thus, it can become more easily triggered than in someone without PTSD.

The anterior cingulate cortex may also play a role in PTSD, as individuals with more active cingulate cortices tend to not respond well to treatments like cognitive behavioral therapy (Martin et al., 2009).

Cognitive structures in the brain may also have an inability to suppress intrusive thoughts and negative emotional memories in PTSD. For example, individuals with PTSD have less responsive brain areas associated with executive function, such as the prefrontal cortex, and hyperactivity in regions correlated with fear, like the amygdala (Shin, 2006). The magnitude of reactivity is also associated with symptom severity. Thus, a more active amygdala and a less active prefrontal cortex are related to having more severe PTSD symptoms (Shin, 2006). The hippocampus may also function differently leading to problems with memory, but more research needs to be conducted to confirm these results.

Neurotransmitters may be out of balance in PTSD as well. Glutamate, the brain's most abundant excitatory neurotransmitter, is involved in learning associated with the hippocampus as well as the processing of stressful emotions in the amygdala. Too much glutamate or erratic signaling could lead to increased activity in these regions of the brain (Averill *et al.*, 2017). Norepinephrine (a neurotransmitter and stress hormone) may also be abnormal in PTSD. Normally, norepinephrine is secreted during acute stress to raise heart rate and blood pressure, but in PTSD, levels of norepinephrine appear to remain elevated after the triggering event (Southwick *et al.*, 1999).

The HPA axis stress pathway may function differently in PTSD, but results have been inconsistent across studies (Dunlop and Wong, 2019). Some studies have shown a decrease in cortisol concentrations (produced by the HPA axis during stress) in individuals with PTSD compared with controls, while other studies have shown no significant difference between groups (Klaassens *et al.*, 2012). Individuals with PTSD may also have altered levels of corticotropin-releasing factor and/or adrenocorticotrophic hormone, which are both produced during HPA axis activation (de Kloet *et al.*, 2007; Carpenter *et al.*, 2007).

There is also likely a genetic component to PTSD. In particular, genes that interact with early life stress could be of great importance. The expression of the FK506 binding protein 5 gene is induced by acute trauma and associated with developing PTSD (Sarapas *et al.*, 2011; Watkins *et al.*, 2016). There are likely many more genes at play, and further studies will help define the exact mechanisms underlying PTSD.

Yoga and meditation for PTSD

Multiple studies have examined the effect of yoga and meditation practice on symptoms of PTSD. A review of 10 studies, which included 643 participants, found that meditation interventions of mindfulness-based stress reduction, yoga and other styles of meditation appeared to be effective in reducing PTSD and depressive symptoms (Hilton *et al.*, 2017). Yet, another review of seven randomized control studies of yoga interventions for people with PTSD found that there was wide variation in effectiveness (Sciarrino *et al.*, 2017).

Despite the range of findings among the general population, meditation interventions tailored for military veterans with PTSD have consistently shown positive results. Scientists from the Naval Medical University in China examined the efficacy of mindfulness meditation in the treatment of military-related PTSD (Sun *et al.*, 2021). The review included 1,326 participants across 19 selected articles. The results revealed that mindfulness meditation worked well in alleviating military-related PTSD symptoms when compared with the control conditions.

To better understand how contemplative practices impact veterans, scientists from the University of Hawai'i partnered with the nonprofit Warriors at Ease to conduct a study examining veterans' perceptions of the benefits, barriers and motivations for practicing trauma-sensitive yoga (Cushing, Braun and Alden, 2018). Warriors at Ease offers trauma-sensitive, military-culture informed mind–body practices to veterans. The scientists conducted interviews with nine veterans to find out more about how trauma-sensitive yoga was affecting their lives.

Many themes emerged from the interviews; veterans found mental stillness, body awareness and social connection through the yoga intervention. Importantly, the authors also identified multiple barriers to practicing yoga, which included the perceptions that yoga is socially unacceptable for men and not physically challenging (Cushing, Braun and Alden, 2018). Yoga could be made more inclusive for veterans by having more male instructors who are service members or veterans themselves teach the classes. This small change could help alter the perception that strong men don't belong in class (Cushing, Braun and Alden, 2018). Yoga could also be a proactive measure as part of physical activity routines or active duty, instead of being only recommended after trauma.

In a study where the yoga intervention was led by a veteran, scientists found that military-tailored yoga significantly reduced three facets of PTSD, including hyperarousal, flashbacks and avoidance (Cushing *et al.*, 2018). The veterans in the study also showed improved mindfulness, and insomnia and anxiety symptoms. Thus, trauma-sensitive yoga interventions may be an effective adjunctive therapy for treating PTSD.

> **Main takeaways**
> - **Post-traumatic stress disorder** (PTSD) is a trauma- or stress-related disorder that involves persistent mental and emotional stress, sleep disturbances and vivid recall of a stressful experience.
> - Yoga and meditation can reduce symptoms of PTSD.
> - Mindfulness meditation can significantly reduce PTSD symptoms in military veterans. Veterans report feelings of calm, increased bodily awareness and social connection after meditation interventions.
> - Military-tailored yoga can help to decrease hyperarousal, flashbacks and avoidance in veterans with PTSD.

DEPRESSION

Depression is a mental condition that is characterized by feelings of despondency and dejection. It can affect how the person feels, thinks and behaves, including causing persistent feelings of sadness and loss of interest in previously enjoyed activities. Depression can occur due to a variety of reasons, including genetic, environmental, situational and psychological factors.

Depression is the leading cause of disability in the United States for people aged 15–44, affecting roughly 10 percent of US adults, according to the Anxiety and Depression Association of America (ADAA). It is estimated that over 350 million people have some form of depression worldwide (Bridges and Sharma, 2017; Shadrina, Bondarenko and Slominsky, 2018; ADAA, 2022).

People are not born with depression. Instead, there is a trigger or stressful event that sets off a cascade of molecular events leading to the onset of depression. Neuroscientists do not fully understand the mechanisms of depression in the brain, and it is not as simple as one chemical being too low and another being too high (Harvard Health Publishing, 2022). Rather, there are millions (or maybe even billions) of chemical reactions occurring every moment that alter mood and the perception of life. Thus, there is no one cause of depression. Two people may experience similar symptoms but have very different chemical reactions occurring in their brains.

Certain brain regions also play a role in depression. These include areas that help regulate mood, such as the hippocampus, amygdala and thalamus. Neuroimaging studies have shown that the hippocampus, the long-term memory center, is smaller in people with depression. One study of 24 women with a history of recurrent major depression showed that the hippocampi of the depressed women were, on average, 9–13 percent smaller than the hippocampi of the healthy controls (Sheline et al., 1999). Additionally, the more bouts of depression an individual had, the smaller their hippocampus appeared. Chronic stress could play a role in affecting hippocampal size, as stress leads to an increase in the release of cortisol, which, over time, is known to kill neurons.

The amygdala, which is involved in feelings of anger, fear, arousal and pleasure, becomes activated when recalling an emotionally charged memory. Individuals with depression have larger amygdalas than those without depression, suggesting more activity and neural activation (van Eijndhoven et al., 2009). Lastly, the relay station of the brain, the thalamus, is also thought to be altered in depression. Depression could partly result from problems relaying sensory information that is linked to pleasant and unpleasant feelings. Thus, someone with depression may experience unpleasant feelings more often, even when the stimulus is not inherently bad.

Similar to anxiety and PTSD, there are also different genes that make some people more susceptible to depression than others. Twin and family studies have shown that the heritability rate for depression is 37 percent (Shadrina, Bondarenko and Slominsky, 2018). The most commonly studied gene is *SLC6A4*, which regulates the neurotransmitter serotonin (Shadrina, Bondarenko and Slominsky, 2018). Studies suggest that this gene becomes downregulated in depression, leading to less available serotonin at the synapse, the connection between neurons. The commonly prescribed depression medications, serotonin-reuptake inhibitors (SSRIs), increase the amount of serotonin at the synapse. SSRIs work, but not immediately – it usually takes a few weeks to months before symptoms start to improve – and scientists still do not fully understand why increasing serotonin decreases symptoms of depression in many people.

Despite having some effective medications on the market, many individuals choose to not take medications due to the side effects, lack of access or personal choice (Bridges and Sharma, 2017). There is also social stigma around antidepressant medications, and mental health in general, which discourages individuals from seeking treatment. There is a clear need to study and evaluate alterative treatment methods.

Yoga for depression

Mind–body interventions, such as yoga and meditation, are now being tested as treatment options for depression. Although yoga may not significantly reduce symptoms of anxiety, it has been shown to be a helpful tool for depression. Scientists from Jackson State University who reviewed 23 studies examining yoga as an alternative or complementary treatment for depression found that yoga does help to decrease symptoms in both individuals with depression and their caregivers (Bridges and Sharma, 2017). The studies reviewed had small to medium sample sizes ranging from 14 to 136 participants, which limits the power of statistical analysis. Unfortunately, most of the studies did not specify which type of yoga was used as the intervention, so it is unclear if one type of yoga is better than others for treating depression.

> **How much yoga do I need to practice to improve my symptoms of depression?**
> **Short answer:** Practicing yoga two to three times a week may be enough to see improvements.
>
> Scientists from Boston University tested the dosing effect by comparing a high-dose yoga group with a low-dose group in participants with major depressive disorder (Streeter *et al.*, 2017). The high-dose group practiced Iyengar yoga and slow, deep breathing (5 breaths/minute) three times a week for 12 weeks, while the low-dose group practiced twice a week.
>
> Both groups showed a significant decrease in depressive symptoms. Thus, practicing yoga and breath work twice a week is likely to be enough to see a noticeable difference.

EXAMPLE GROUNDED SUN SALUTATION VARIATION FLOW FOR PROMOTING MIND–BODY CONNECTION

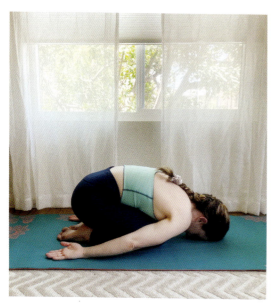

Figure 8.5 Child's pose.

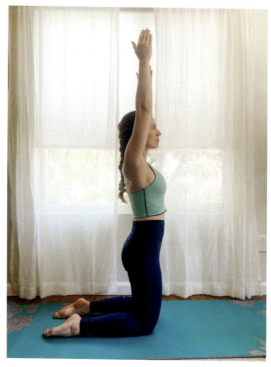

Figure 8.7 Kneeling pose with arms extended overhead.

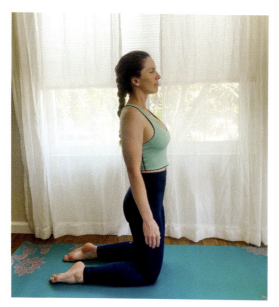

Figure 8.6 Kneeling pose.

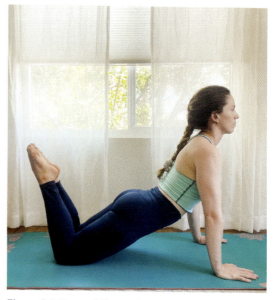

Figure 8.8 Upward-facing dog variation.

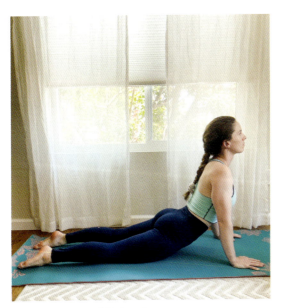

Figure 8.9 Upward-facing dog.

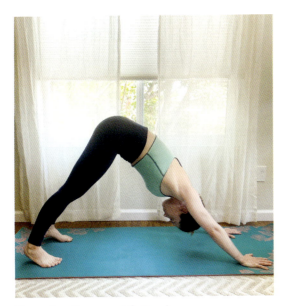

Figure 8.10 Downward-facing dog.

Meditation for depression

There have been several studies conducted on using meditation as a treatment for depression. Scientists from the VA Puget Sound Health Care System in Seattle, Washington examined the meditation literature to see if mindfulness meditation interventions could help treat a variety of psychiatric conditions, including depression (Goldberg et al., 2018). Their review included 12,005 participants from 142 different samples. They found that across all studies, mindfulness showed strong evidence for helping to reduce symptoms of depression. Mindfulness interventions were better than no treatment and other active treatments, as well as equivalent in efficacy as the evidence-based treatments. These results held true at the study follow-ups as well. Taken together, these results strongly suggest that mindfulness-based interventions can be an effective alternative or adjunctive treatment for depression.

Mindfulness meditation interventions have also been shown to be an effective treatment option for older adults (≥65 years old) with depression. Researchers from Saint Louis University conducted a systematic review and meta-analysis of 19 studies that included over 1,000 participants (Reangsing, Rittiwong and Schneider, 2020). Overall, mindfulness meditation interventions improved symptoms of depression. Specifically, interventions that included guided meditation were the most effective at reducing symptoms of depression compared with interventions without. Thus, guided meditation should be included in therapy involving older populations.

Is yoga or meditation better for reducing symptoms of depression?

One study was designed to answer this exact question (Falsafi, 2016). The researcher set up a randomized control trial that consisted of a yoga group, a mindfulness meditation group and a control group in 90 college students who had a diagnosis of depression and/or anxiety. Participants in the yoga and meditation groups received a two-month training, and symptoms of depression and anxiety were measured at baseline, one month, two months and three months later.

The scientist found that symptoms of depression decreased significantly in the yoga and meditation groups from the baseline to the follow-up time points. However, the results did not significantly differ between the yoga and meditation groups. One exception was that the meditation group did show improvements in self-compassion, which was not observed in the yoga group. Thus, meditation and yoga both seem to offer some benefit for those with depression.

Main takeaways
- **Depression** is a mood disorder that is characterized by feelings of despondency and dejection.
- Yoga helps to decrease symptoms of depression in both individuals with depression and their caregivers. Practicing yoga two to three times a week may be enough to see improvements in symptomology.
- There is strong evidence demonstrating that mindfulness meditation can help to reduce symptoms of depression.
- Guided meditation may be the most effective form of meditation for reducing symptoms of depression in adults aged 65 and older.

REFERENCES

Anxiety and Depression Association of America (ADAA), 2022. Anxiety disorders: facts & statistics. Anxiety and Depression Association of America. Available at: https://adaa.org/understanding-anxiety/facts-statistics

Averill, L.A., Purohit, P., Averill, C.L., Boesl, M.A., Krystal, J.H., & Abdallah, C.G., 2017. Glutamate dysregulation and glutamatergic therapeutics for PTSD: evidence from human studies. *Neuroscience Letters*, 649, pp.147-155.

Bhasin, M.K., Dusek, J.A., Chang, B., Joseph, M.G., et al., 2013. Relaxation response induces temporal transcriptome changes in energy metabolism, insulin secretion and inflammatory pathways. *PLoS ONE*, 8(5), e62817.

Blanck, P., Perleth, S., Heidenreich, T., Kröger, P., et al., 2018. Effects of mindfulness exercises as stand-alone intervention on symptoms of anxiety and depression: systematic review and meta-analysis. *Behaviour Research and Therapy*, 102, pp.25-35.

Bridges, L., & Sharma, M., 2017. The efficacy of yoga as a form of treatment for depression. *Journal of Evidence-Based Complementary & Alternative Medicine*, 22(4), pp.1017-1028.

Buchanan, T.W., Bagley, S.L., Stansfield, R.B., & Preston, S.D., 2012. The empathic, physiological resonance of stress. *Social Neuroscience*, 7(2), pp.191-201.

Carpenter, L.L., Carvalho, J.P., Tyrka, A.R., Wier, L.M., et al., 2007. Decreased adrenocorticotropic hormone and cortisol responses to stress in healthy adults reporting significant childhood maltreatment. *Biological Psychiatry*, 62(10), pp.1080-1087.

Cramer, H., Lauche, R., Anheyer, D., Pilkington, K., et al., 2018. Yoga for anxiety: a systematic review and meta-analysis of randomized controlled trials. *Depression and Anxiety*, 35(9), pp.830-843.

Cushing, R.E., Braun, K.L., Alden, S.W., & Katz, A.R., 2018. Military-tailored yoga for veterans with post-traumatic stress disorder. *Military Medicine*, 183(5-6), pp.e223-e231.

Cushing, R.E., Braun, K.L., & Alden, S., 2018. A qualitative study exploring yoga in veterans with PTSD symptoms. *International Journal of Yoga Therapy*, 28(1), pp.63-70.

de Kloet, C.S., Vermetten, E., Geuze, E., Lentjes, E.G.W.M., et al., 2007. Elevated plasma corticotrophin-releasing hormone levels in veterans with posttraumatic stress disorder. *Progress in Brain Research*, 167, pp.287-291.

Djalilova, D.M., Schulz, P.S., Berger, A.M., Case, A.J., Kupzyk, K.A., & Ross A.C., 2018. Impact of yoga on inflammatory biomarkers: a systematic review. *Biological Research for Nursing*, 21(2), pp.198-209.

Dunlop, B.W., & Wong, A., 2019. The hypothalamic-pituitary-adrenal axis in PTSD: pathophysiology and treatment interventions. *Progress in Neuro-Psychopharmacology and Biological Psychiatry*, 89, pp.361-379.

Epel, E.S., Blackburn, E.H., Lin, J., Dhabhar, F.S., Adler, N.E., Morrow, J.D., et al., 2004. Accelerated telomere shortening in response to life stress. *Proceedings of the National Academy of Sciences*, 101(49), pp.17312-17315.

Falkenberg, R.I., Eising, C., & Peters, M.L., 2018. Yoga and immune system functioning: a systematic review of randomized controlled trials. *Journal of Behavioral Medicine*, 41(4), pp.467-482.

Falsafi, N., 2016. A randomized controlled trial of mindfulness versus yoga. *Journal of the American Psychiatric Nurses Association*, 22(6), pp.483-497.

Fang, C.Y., Reibel, D.K., Longacre, M.L., Rosenzweig, S., Campbell, D.E., & Douglas, S.D., 2010. Enhanced psychosocial well-being following participation in a mindfulness-based stress reduction program is associated with increased natural killer cell activity. *The*

Journal of Alternative and Complementary Medicine, 16(5), pp.531–538.

Goldberg, S.B., Tucker, R.P., Greene, P.A., Davidson, R.J., et al., 2018. Mindfulness-based interventions for psychiatric disorders: a systematic review and meta-analysis. *Clinical Psychology Review*, 59, pp.52–60.

Gosain, A., Jones, S.B., Shankar, R., Gamelli, R.L., & DiPietro, L., 2006. Norepinephrine modulates the inflammatory and proliferative phases of wound healing. *The Journal of Trauma: Injury, Infection, and Critical Care*, 60(4), pp.736–744.

Goyal, M., Singh, S., Sibinga, E.M.S., Gould, N.F., et al., 2014. Meditation programs for psychological stress and well-being. *JAMA Internal Medicine*, 174(3), p.357.

Harvard Health Publishing, 2022. What causes depression? Available at: https://www.health.harvard.edu/mind-and-mood/what-causes-depression

Hearon, C.M., & Dinenno, F.A., 2015. Regulation of skeletal muscle blood flow during exercise in ageing humans. *The Journal of Physiology*, 594(8), pp.2261–2273.

Hilton, L., Maher, A.R., Colaiaco, B., Apaydin, E., et al., 2017. Meditation for posttraumatic stress: systematic review and meta-analysis. *Psychological Trauma: Theory, Research, Practice, and Policy*, 9(4), pp.453–460.

Hoge, E.A., Bui, E., Marques, L., Metcalf, C.A., et al., 2013. Randomized controlled trial of mindfulness meditation for generalized anxiety disorder. *The Journal of Clinical Psychiatry*, 74(08), pp.786–792.

Hoge, E.A., Bui, E., Mete, M., Dutton, M.A., Baker, A.W., & Simon, N.M., 2022. Mindfulness-based stress reduction vs escitalopram for the treatment of adults with anxiety disorders: a randomized clinical trial. *JAMA Psychiatry*. Doi:10.1001/jamapsychiatry.2022.3679.

Idriss, H.T., & Naismith, J.H., 2000. TNF alpha and the TNF receptor superfamily: structure-function relationship(s). *Microscopy Research and Technique*, 50(3), pp.184–195.

Kiecolt-Glaser, J.K., Christian, L., Preston, H., Houts, C.R., et al., 2010. Stress, inflammation, and yoga practice. *Psychosomatic Medicine*, 72(2), pp.113–121.

Kiecolt-Glaser, J.K., Bennett, J.M., Andridge, R., Peng, J., et al., 2014. Yoga's impact on inflammation, mood, and fatigue in breast cancer survivors: a randomized controlled trial. *Journal of Clinical Oncology*, 32(10), pp.1040–1049.

Kirschbaum, C., Pirke, K.-M., & Hellhammer, D.H., 1993. The "Trier Social Stress Test" – a tool for investigating psychobiological stress responses in a laboratory setting. *Neuropsychobiology*, 28(1–2), pp.76–81.

Klaassens, E.R., Giltay, E.J., Cuijpers, P., van Veen, T., & Zitman, F.G., 2012. Adulthood trauma and HPA-axis functioning in healthy subjects and PTSD patients: a meta-analysis. *Psychoneuroendocrinology*, 37(3), pp.317–331.

Lemay, V., Hoolahan, J., & Buchanan, A., 2019. Impact of a yoga and meditation intervention on students' stress and anxiety levels. *American Journal of Pharmaceutical Education*, 83(5), p.7001.

Liu, Y.-Z., Wang, Y.-X., & Jiang, C.-L., 2017. Inflammation: the common pathway of stress-related diseases. *Frontiers in Human Neuroscience*, 11, p.316.

Lopez-Castejon, G., & Brough, D., 2011. Understanding the mechanism of IL-1β secretion. *Cytokine Growth Factor Reviews*, 22(4), pp.189–195.

Luan, Y.Y., & Yao, Y.M., 2018. The clinical significance and potential role of c-reactive protein in chronic inflammatory and neurodegenerative diseases. *Frontiers in Immunology*, 9, 1302.

Lupien, S.J., McEwen, B.S., Gunnar, M.R., & Heim, C., 2009. Effects of stress throughout the lifespan on the brain, behaviour and cognition. *Nature Reviews Neuroscience*, 10(6), pp.434–445.

Martin, E.I., Ressler, K.J., Binder, E., & Nemeroff, C.B., 2009. The neurobiology of anxiety disorders: brain imaging, genetics, and psychoneuroendocrinology. *Psychiatric Clinics of North America*, 32(3), pp.549–575.

Matiz, A., Fabbro, F., Paschetto, A., Cantone, D., Paolone, A.R., & Crescentini, C., 2020. Positive impact of mindfulness meditation on mental health of female teachers during the COVID-19 outbreak in Italy. *International Journal of Environmental Research and Public Health*, 17(18), p.6450.

Pace, T.W.W., Negi, L.T., Dodson-Lavelle, B., Ozawa-de Silva, B., et al., 2013. Engagement with cognitively-based compassion training is associated with reduced salivary C-reactive protein from before to after training in foster care program adolescents. *Psychoneuroendocrinology*, 38(2), pp.294–299.

Reangsing, C., Rittiwong, T., & Schneider, J.K., 2020. Effects of mindfulness meditation interventions on depression in older adults: a meta-analysis. *Aging & Mental Health*, 25(7), pp.1181–1190.

Richter-Levin, G., & Sandi, C., 2021. Title: "Labels matter: is it stress or is it trauma?" *Translational Psychiatry*, 11(1), p.385.

Rosenkranz, M.A., Davidson, R.J., MacCoon, D.G., Sheridan, J.F., Kalin, N.H., & Lutz, A., 2013. A comparison of mindfulness-based stress reduction and an active control in modulation of neurogenic inflammation. *Brain, Behavior, and Immunity*, 27, pp.174–184.

Sarapas, C., Cai, G., Bierer, L.M., Golier, J.A., et al., 2011. Genetic markers for PTSD risk and resilience among survivors of the World Trade Center attacks. *Disease Markers*, 30(2–3), pp.101–110.

Schutte, N.S., & Malouff, J.M., 2014. A meta-analytic review of the effects of mindfulness meditation on telomerase activity. *Psychoneuroendocrinology*, 42, pp.45–48.

Sciarrino, N.A, DeLucia, C., O'Brien, K., & McAdams, K., 2017. Assessing the effectiveness of yoga as a complementary and alternative treatment for post-traumatic stress disorder: a review and synthesis. *The Journal of Alternative and Complementary Medicine*, 23(10), pp.747–755.

Shadrina, M., Bondarenko, E.A., & Slominsky, P.A., 2018. Genetics factors in major depression disease. *Frontiers in Psychiatry*, 9, p.334.

Sheline, Y.I., Sanghavi, M., Mintun, M.A., & Gado, M.H., 1999. Depression duration but not age predicts hippocampal volume loss in medically healthy women with recurrent major depression. *The Journal of Neuroscience*, 19(12), pp.5034-5043.

Shin, L.M., 2006. Amygdala, medial prefrontal cortex, and hippocampal function in PTSD. *Annals of the New York Academy of Sciences*, 1071(1), pp.67-79.

Southwick, S.M., Paige, S., Morgan, C.A., Bremner, J.D., Krystal, J.H., & Charney, D.S., 1999. Neurotransmitter alterations in PTSD: catecholamines and serotonin. *Seminars in Clinical Neuropsychiatry*, 4(4), pp.242-248.

Streeter, C.C., Gerbarg, P.L., Whitfield, T.H., Owen, L., *et al.*, 2017. Treatment of major depressive disorder with Iyengar yoga and coherent breathing: a randomized controlled dosing study. *Alternative and Complementary Therapies*, 23(6), pp.236-243.

Sun, L.-N., Gu, J.-W., Huang, L.-J., Shang, Z.-L., *et al.*, 2021. Military-related posttraumatic stress disorder and mindfulness meditation: a systematic review and meta-analysis. *Chinese Journal of Traumatology*, 24(4), pp.221-230.

Tanaka T., Narazaki, M., & Kishimoto, T., 2014. IL-6 in inflammation, immunity, and disease. *Cold Spring Harbor Perspective Biology*, 4;6(10), a016295.

van Eijndhoven, P. van Wingen, G., van Oijen, K., Rijpkema, M., *et al.*, 2009. Amygdala volume marks the acute state in the early course of depression. *Biological Psychiatry*, 65(9), pp.812-818.

Venkatesh, H.N., Ravish, H., Wilma Delphine Silvia, C.R., & Srinivas, H., 2020. Molecular signature of the immune response to yoga therapy in stress-related chronic disease conditions: an insight. *International Journal of Yoga*, 13(1), pp.9-17.

Vollbehr, N.K., Bartels-Velthuis, A.A., Nauta, M.H., Castelein, S., *et al.*, 2018. Hatha yoga for acute, chronic and/or treatment-resistant mood and anxiety disorders: a systematic review and meta-analysis. *PLoS ONE*, 13(10), e0204925.

Watkins, L.E., Han, S., Harpaz-Rotem, I., Mota, N.P., *et al.*, 2016. FKBP5 polymorphisms, childhood abuse, and PTSD symptoms: results from the National Health and Resilience in Veterans study. *Psychoneuroendocrinology*, 69, pp.98-105.

Weaver, L.L., & Darragh, A.R., 2015. Systematic review of yoga interventions for anxiety reduction among children and adolescents. *The American Journal of Occupational Therapy*, 69(6), 6906180070p1-9.

Wolkowitz, O.M., Mellon, S.H., Epel, E.S., Lin J., *et al.*, 2011. Resting leukocyte telomerase activity is elevated in major depression and predicts treatment response. *Molecular Psychiatry*, 17(2), pp.164-172.

CHAPTER 9

The Effect of Yoga and Meditation on the Brain

Neurological Conditions, Chronic Pain and Addiction

The brain is the body's control center, and it can be altered by traumatic injury and illness. Neurological conditions arise when the brain, spinal cord or nerves become injured or impaired, affecting function and leading to a range of symptoms. In this chapter, we'll cover some of the most common neurological disorders, including traumatic brain injury, stroke, multiple sclerosis and Alzheimer's disease. Many of these conditions include the symptom of chronic pain, which we'll examine to explore how yoga and meditation can help. Other conditions relating to chronic pain, such as arthritis and addiction, will also be discussed as there is convincing evidence that contemplative practices can make a positive impact.

TRAUMATIC BRAIN INJURY

Traumatic brain injury (TBI) is an injury to the head that causes damage to the brain. It can be the result of a fall, a blow to the head or even an object penetrating the skull (remember Mr. Gage from Chapter 3?). TBI affects brain function, and the injury can damage one area of the brain or be more diffuse, impacting multiple brain regions. Roughly 13.5 million Americans live with a disability due to TBI, according to the American Association of Neurological Surgeons (AANS, 2020).

The most common type of TBI is a closed brain injury, which occurs when there is a rapid change in movement of the head causing bruising or tearing of brain tissue and blood vessels. A closed brain injury can be the result of a car accident, sporting mishap or a fall. Concussions are a common type of closed brain TBI.

When the skull hits an object, the brain slams into the skull at the site of impact, resulting in an initial injury called a coup injury. A secondary injury can also occur when the brain bounces back, hitting the opposite part of the skull; this is called a contrecoup injury (Figure 9.1). Thus, even if someone's head collided with an object in the front, they might also experience a TBI in the back of the brain. If the occipital lobe received damage during a contrecoup injury, then neurons might fire sporadically causing the person to "see stars" for a period after the injury.

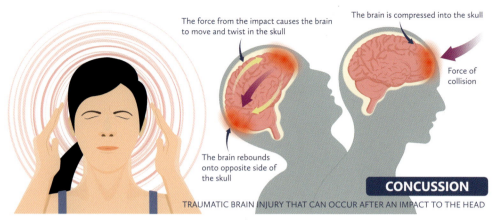

Figure 9.1 Traumatic brain injury can involve a coup and contrecoup injury.

A person who experiences a contrecoup injury might also have a diffuse axonal injury. In this type of brain injury, the axons of the neurons are torn due to the strong force of the brain shifting inside the skull (Figure 9.2). A diffuse axonal injury often results in coma and injury to multiple parts of the brain.

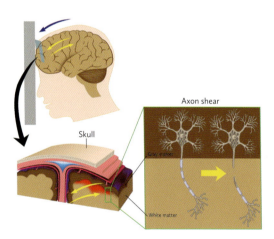

Figure 9.2 A diffuse axonal injury where the axons of the neurons are torn.

Although a TBI can occur immediately after an accident, called a primary injury, a secondary brain injury can occur hours or even days after the event. Secondary brain injuries usually happen on a microscopic level and involve changes to the cells or blood vessels that result in further damage. One of the most well-known examples of secondary brain injury occurred in 2009 when actress Natasha Richardson fell while skiing in Canada. She was not wearing a helmet at the time. Initially, she reportedly felt fine, but developed a severe headache an hour or two after the fall, which prompted a trip to the hospital. She unfortunately passed away two days later after developing an epidural hematoma, a type of brain bleed where blood accumulates between the skull and the thicker outer covering of the brain. Her story drew national attention to the importance of TBI treatment and prevention (Stump, 2009).

There is a broad spectrum of severity of traumatic brain injuries, which can range from a mild contusion to a life-threatening event. Depending on the severity and type of TBI, individuals may experience a range of symptoms, including cognitive defects, issues with movement, changes in the senses, difficulty speaking, impaired social skills, and personality changes, among others (Johns Hopkins Medicine, 2022). TBI is often invisible to others, so survivors can feel isolated, misunderstood and have difficulty finding compassionate care.

Scientists believe that once brain cells are damaged or destroyed, it may be difficult for them to heal or regenerate. However, the human brain is malleable. In some cases, connections between neurons can be rerouted to uninjured areas of the brain to restore function (Johns Hopkins Medicine, 2022). For those with severe injuries, recovery can require a lifetime of rehabilitation, so finding effective treatments is imperative. Contemplative practices are an effective tool in reducing symptomology and improving quality of life in many TBI survivors.

Yoga and meditation for TBI

Yoga and meditation have been shown to improve symptoms of mild TBI across many studies. Researchers from the University of Connecticut reviewed 20 studies with a total of 539 participants and found that meditation, yoga and mindfulness-based interventions can significantly improve mental and physical health, quality of life and cognitive performance while decreasing symptoms of fatigue and depression in people with mild brain injuries (Acabchuk *et al.*, 2020).

The LoveYourBrain Foundation, based in Vermont, is one of the leading organizations offering yoga, meditation, community connection and education to those who have experienced a TBI. It was founded by professional snowboarder Kevin Pearce, who sustained a major TBI while training for the 2010 Winter Olympics. Kevin Pearce, along with his brother Adam Pearce, decided to create a science- and community-based six-week yoga and meditation program to help others who have experienced a TBI.

A few academic studies have been conducted on the impact of the LoveYourBrain Yoga program on TBI survivors and their caregivers. One large study (1,563 participants) showed that participating in the LoveYourBrain program led to a significant improvement in perceived quality of life, well-being and cognition (Donnelly *et al.*, 2019). Additionally, TBI survivors were able to better regulate their levels of anxiety, anger, stress and impulsivity after the yoga program. Caregivers, who also often experience high levels of stress, were found to have improvements in physical and psychological health after participating in the program as well.

In a separate qualitative study, researchers interviewed LoveYourBrain Yoga program participants and found that TBI survivors and their caregivers felt a better sense of belonging, increased community integration, improved physical health, a greater ability to self-regulate and increased resilience (Donnelly, Goldberg and Fournier, 2019).

Tips for teaching someone who has experienced a TBI

- Use simple, slow and repeated movements, as people with TBI sometimes process information and instructions at a different pace.
- Repeat cues often.
- Create a safe space in the studio that is welcoming for all. Remember that people who have experienced a TBI often feel isolated from the community, so try to make an extra effort to be inclusive. Additionally, dimming the lights and keeping noise to a minimum can help people feel more comfortable.
- Carefully instruct the position of the head during movements to avoid neck strain. Be aware that some individuals may have received specific instructions about head position from their care provider.
- Demonstrate movements and sequences when possible. It can be easier for people to follow, especially if the position is new to them.
- Use props and demonstrate how to properly use them. Props can be valuable tools in enabling proper positioning and support of the body.

Adapted with permission from LoveYourBrain.

> **Main takeaways**
> - **Traumatic brain injury** (TBI) is an injury to the head that causes damage to the brain.
> - The most common type of TBI is a closed brain injury, which occurs when there is a rapid change in movement of the head causing bruising or tearing of brain tissue and blood vessels.
> - Yoga and meditation can improve quality of life, cognition, fatigue and depression. These practices can also increase resilience and the ability to self-regulate.

STROKE

Strokes are one of the leading causes of long-term disability in the United States, and roughly 800,000 Americans experience a stroke every year, according to the Centers for Disease Control and Prevention (CDC, 2022a). A **stroke** occurs when part of the brain stops receiving blood flow. There are two main types of stroke: 1) hemorrhagic stroke, which occurs when a blood vessel breaks open; and 2) ischemic stroke, when a blood vessel becomes blocked (Figure 9.3). The lack of oxygen to brain tissue can cause damage or cell death. Roughly 87 percent of strokes are ischemic strokes.

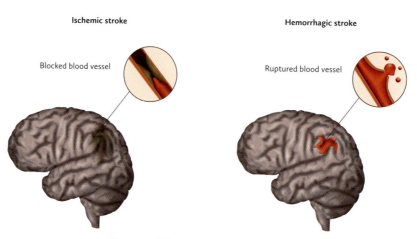

Figure 9.3 The two main types of stroke.

Strokes can occur in any part of the brain; thus, the resulting symptoms of a stroke can vary dramatically depending on the site of the injury. For example, one person may have trouble speaking whereas another person may experience problems with memory. Strokes can also affect movement and lead to difficulty with balance.

The field of neuroscience has a long history of examining the brain changes that occur after a stroke. Before the invention of neuroimaging techniques, neuroscientists would study the brains of stroke patients to see what happened to their behavior when certain areas of the brain were destroyed due to the lack of blood flow.

Will a headstand improve blood flow to the brain?

It is often suggested in yoga classes that performing a headstand improves blood flow to the brain; however, this is not the case.

Blood flow to the brain is highly regulated, and performing a headstand will not significantly increase or decrease flow, according to a recent study (Minvaleev et al., 2019). In the study, researchers measured the blood flow of the internal carotid artery using ultrasound in 20 people performing a headstand. They found that at the start of a headstand there is actually a decrease in the blood flow to the brain, followed by a return to baseline values. This result is likely due to the mechanism of autoregulation, which keeps the flow of blood to the brain consistent, regardless of body position. Although the initial change in body position did cause a change in blood flow, the body quickly adjusted to keep blood flow consistent.

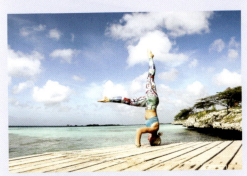

Figure 9.4 Headstand does not increase blood flow to the brain.
Source: Annemiek Smegen on Unsplash.

Yoga for stroke

There have been very few studies examining how yoga can improve movement and quality of life in stroke survivors. Scientists from Glasgow Caledonian University in the UK reviewed two randomized control trials with 72 participants and found that yoga improved memory but none of the physical, emotional, social or communication aspects of recovery (Lawrence et al., 2017). Unfortunately, the data from these two studies did not confirm or refute the effectiveness of yoga as a therapy for stroke. Additionally, both studies were low quality and at high risk for bias. However, the authors stress that yoga should still be investigated as a potentially useful tool for stroke rehabilitation.

Another review of five randomized control trials conducted by researchers at Monash University in Australia found that yoga improved balance and quality of life, although these results were not significant (Thayabaranathan et al., 2017). However, yoga did significantly help decrease symptoms of anxiety and depression when compared with the control group, suggesting mental health benefits.

Focusing more on the psychological benefits of practicing yoga, researchers from the University of South Australia interviewed nine stroke survivors after they completed a ten-week yoga and meditation intervention (Garrett, Immink and Hillier, 2011). Overall, the participants felt calmer and more connected with their bodies after the yoga and meditation program. They also reported feeling improved strength and ability to move. The study highlights that although the current evidence behind yoga as a treatment for stroke may not be strong, yoga could still be a helpful tool for improving psychological and physical health.

Chair yoga is a popular form of adaptive yoga in which postures are performed either while seated or with the use of a chair or wheelchair. Chair yoga is more accessible and adaptable than mat-based yoga. Importantly, chair yoga removes the physical challenges that some people experience with other forms of yoga.

**CHAIR-BASED YOGA EXERCISES
FOR STROKE SURVIVORS**

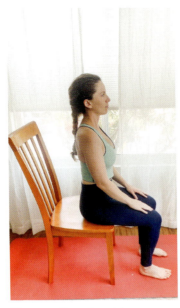

Figure 9.5 Seated position on the chair.

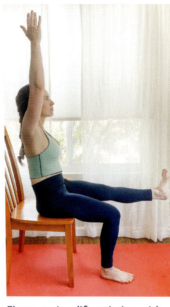

Figure 9.7 Leg lift variation with opposite arm and leg lifted.

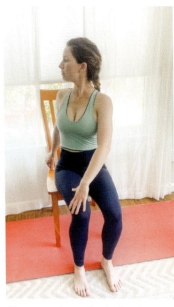

Figure 9.9 Seated spinal twist.

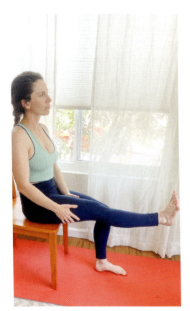

Figure 9.6 Leg lift.

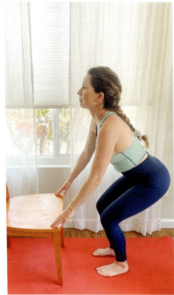

Figure 9.8 Chair pose with arms used for balance.

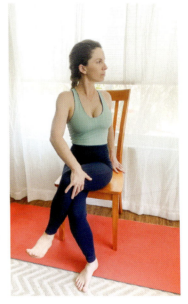

Figure 9.10 Seated spinal twist variation.

Meditation for stroke

Meditation can reduce the risk of stroke by decreasing blood pressure and stress (Larkin, 2000), yet few studies have looked at the effect of meditation on improving post-stroke symptoms.

One pilot study examined how a two-week meditation program could affect quality of life and spasticity in stroke survivors (Wathugala et al., 2019). Spasticity is an abnormal contraction of the muscles, which can interfere with movement. In the study, ten participants listened to short mindfulness meditation recordings, filled out questionnaires and kept a journal. Participants reported improvements in spasticity, energy and productivity, suggesting that even a short meditation intervention could help those recovering from a stroke.

Main takeaways
- A **stroke** occurs when part of the brain stops receiving blood.
- The two main types of stroke are hemorrhagic stroke (when a blood vessel breaks open) and ischemic stroke (when a blood vessel becomes blocked).
- Headstand will not improve blood flow to the brain.
- Yoga interventions may help to improve memory, strength, movement, balance and quality of life as well as decrease symptoms of anxiety and depression.
- Meditation is an effective method for decreasing the risk of stroke and could help to reduce issues with spasticity that can occur after a stroke.

MULTIPLE SCLEROSIS

Multiple sclerosis (MS) is the most common disabling neurological disease affecting young adults aged 20–40 years old, and women are more commonly affected than men. MS is an autoimmune disease of the central nervous system (brain and spinal cord) where the immune system mistakenly attacks the protective myelin sheath around the nerve fibers in the central nervous system (Figure 9.11).

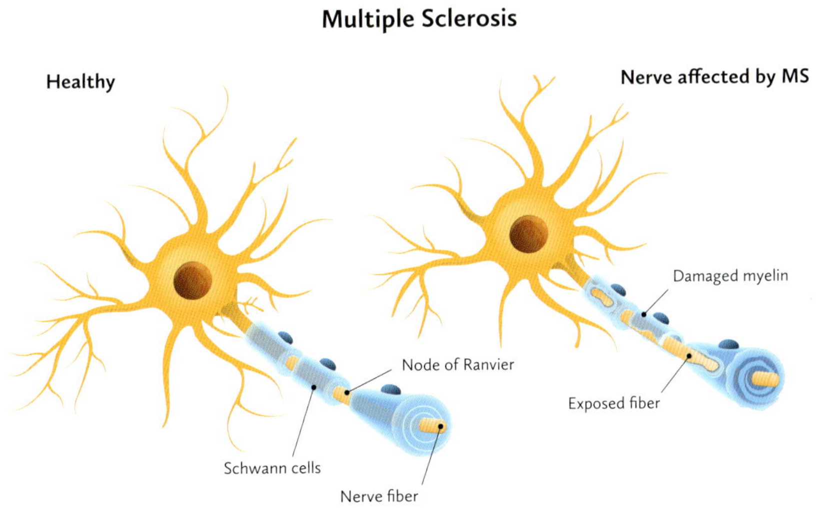

Figure 9.11 The myelin sheath around nerves is affected in multiple sclerosis.

When the myelin is broken down, the electrical signals cannot be transmitted quickly enough, and communication errors occur. This condition can cause communication problems between the brain and the rest of the body, resulting in weakness, numbness, tingling, chronic pain, tremors, vision problems, fatigue and other symptoms. The symptoms of MS can vary widely from person to person depending on the amount of nerve damage, and the location and type of nerves that are affected. Some people may have very few or subtle symptoms while others struggle to move independently or at all.

While there are four main types of MS, the most common form of MS is called relapsing-remitting. Affected individuals experience periods of symptoms that last days or weeks (relapses) and then extended periods of time when their symptoms improve or resolve (remissions). The ups and downs can be physically challenging and mentally taxing. While the forms of MS can change throughout a patient's lifetime, approximately 85 percent of patients with MS are initially diagnosed as having the relapsing-remitting form (National Multiple Sclerosis Society, 2022).

Yoga for multiple sclerosis
Yoga holds promise for the treatment of MS as it can improve fatigue, mood, flexibility and range of motion. Since the symptoms of MS may include issues with balance and coordination, adaptive yoga may be a great option. Adaptive yoga adjusts the type and style of yoga to the individual, to accommodate changing needs and abilities. The goal of a yoga class for someone with MS is to increase or maintain range of motion and flexibility while preventing injury.

Tips for teaching students with multiple sclerosis
- The physical abilities of people with MS may vary from day to day, so check in with students to learn more about their needs and abilities at the beginning of each class.
- Exercise can raise the body's core temperature, which can aggravate MS symptoms. Suggest movements that are slow, calming and restorative over complicated sequences.
- Offer variations to accommodate different levels of ability.
- Create an environment that encourages people to listen to their bodies.
- Combine postures with breathing exercises to bring awareness to the breath to increase relaxation.
- Movements that require frequent ups and downs, such as a sun salutation, can be difficult for those with MS. Instead, focus the practice on staying at one level or slowly transition between different heights and levels.

CHAIR-BASED YOGA EXERCISES FOR INDIVIDUALS WITH MULTIPLE SCLEROSIS

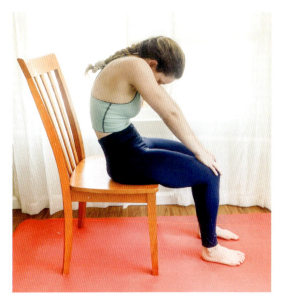

Figure 9.12 Seated cat pose.

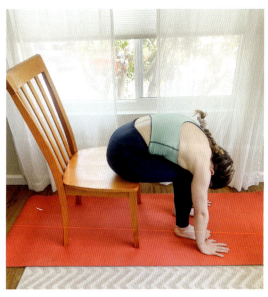

Figure 9.14 Forward fold.

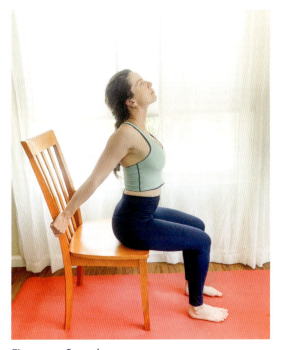

Figure 9.13 Seated cow pose.

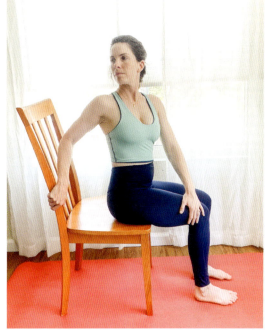

Figure 9.15 Spinal twist.

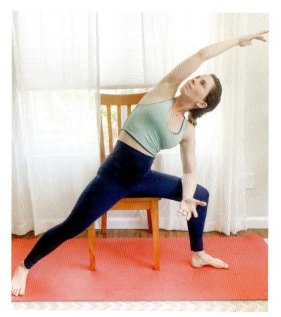

Figure 9.16 Seated extended side angle.

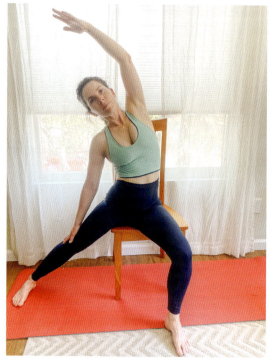

Figure 9.18 Warrior II side stretch variation.

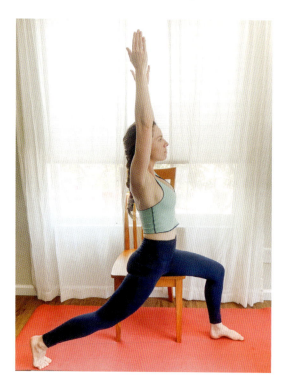

Figure 9.17 Crescent lunge.

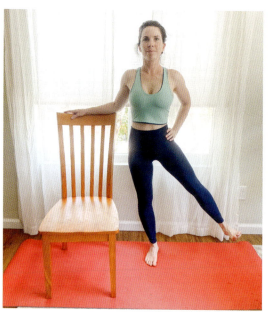

Figure 9.19 Assisted leg lift.

Meditation for multiple sclerosis

The unpredictability of the disease, and ongoing treatments for MS, pose many unique challenges. Patients often need to stay still inside a loud MRI machine for brain scans that can be stressful and last hours. Stress can aggravate symptoms of MS, making these situations even worse.

Researchers from the University of Melbourne, Australia reviewed 12 studies looking at the promise of meditation as an intervention for people with MS and found that meditation can help to improve quality of life and coping skills (Levin et al., 2014). Another study conducted by scientists from the Università Cattolica del Sacro Cuore in Italy and Harvard University with 139 participants found that an online mindfulness meditation intervention helped improve quality of life and lowered symptoms of depression, anxiety and sleep problems in patients more than in the psychoeducation control group (Cavalera et al., 2018). The two-month mindfulness intervention was based on the traditional mindfulness-based stress reduction (MBSR) protocol developed by Jon Kabat-Zinn and adapted to be specific to MS. For example, the authors incorporated music meditations and discussions about MS symptoms acceptance. Despite the immediate benefits of the intervention after eight weeks, the groups were not significantly different at the six-month follow-up. This finding suggests that mindfulness meditation must be practiced consistently to experience beneficial effects.

Main takeaways
- **Multiple sclerosis** (MS) is an autoimmune disease of the central nervous system where the immune system mistakenly attacks the protective myelin sheath around the nerve fibers.
- Yoga can improve fatigue, mood, flexibility and range of motion. Chair yoga is an accessible form of yoga that can be adapted to the individual.
- Meditation can help to improve quality of life and coping skills in those with MS. It may also help to reduce stress, although the benefits may not last if the practice is discontinued.

Relaxation meditation with a focus on the breath

Find your way to a comfortable position. This can be lying down or perhaps sitting up in a chair. Whatever feels best for you in this moment.
Start to bring your attention to the breath. Observe the natural breath and relax into the natural rhythm that the breath offers. Notice how the breath enters and exits the body. Smooth. Effortless.
Allow the arms and legs to relax, letting go of any tension in the limbs.
Now, increase your awareness with the contact points of your body on the floor or the chair. Notice how your body is interacting with and being held by the surrounding environment.
Bring the attention back to the breath and feel as it enters and exits the nostrils. Follow the flow of the breath in and the flow of the breath out.

ALZHEIMER'S DISEASE

Alzheimer's disease is an eventually fatal dementia with no effective treatment options. Although Alzheimer's is common, it is not a normal part of aging. Alzheimer's causes the loss of function or death of neurons in multiple brain regions that leads to memory loss and the inability to hold a conversation or be aware of the environment. Despite decades of research, over 95 percent of Alzheimer's disease cases have no known origin. However, early detection and intervention can help to slow the neurodegeneration.

Age is the biggest risk factor for Alzheimer's, and there is strong evidence that genetics plays a role (Kunkle et al., 2019). Other factors, such as diet, education and exercise, may influence the development of Alzheimer's as well.

There are two main biomarkers that are associated with the disease. The first is amyloid beta plaques, which are pieces of amyloid precursor protein, a type of membrane protein found in many tissues and in neuron synapses. Amyloid beta protein can build up in the brain to become plaques in the spaces surrounding neurons. Although scientists don't fully understand the mechanism, it appears that amyloid beta plaques lead to cell death, changes in metabolism and an increase in inflammation in the brain. These factors can lead to abnormal functioning of the brain. However, some people develop amyloid beta plaques and do not develop Alzheimer's.

The other notable biomarker is called tau, which is a structural protein inside neurons. In Alzheimer's, tau starts to form abnormal clumps called tangles, which are thought to damage the structure of the neurons. This process likely leads to poorly functioning neurons and neuron death.

These biomarkers can be used to determine the stage of the disease, which can help doctors to determine the best way to treat Alzheimer's. Many clinical trials are on-going to test possible treatment options. One drug called CMS121 has been developed and studied by Salk Institute scientists over the last fifteen years. CMS121, which is derived from a natural chemical found in strawberries, reverses signs of aging in the brain and prevents the memory loss associated with Alzheimer's in mice (Ates et al., 2020). The drug is currently undergoing clinical trials to test its effectiveness in humans.

There is also a brain-breach theory of Alzheimer's that involves one of the brain's top defense systems: the **blood–brain barrier**. The blood–brain barrier is a filter between the brain's blood vessels and the brain tissue, and it protects the brain against bacteria, viruses and toxins that could cause a brain infection or damage, while letting in important nutrients.

Researchers have found that stress can make the blood–brain barrier "leaky" (Friedman et al., 1996). The blood–brain barrier also becomes leaky with age, which allows proteins, like albumin, to enter the brain (Senatorov et al., 2019). These changes lead to increased inflammation, abnormal neuronal activity and cognitive decline, which are all indicated in Alzheimer's. The same group of researchers found that giving mice drugs that protected the barrier blocked albumin proteins from entering the brain, reduced inflammation and improved cognition. They suspect that problems with this filter could cause all kinds of neurological conditions, including Alzheimer's.

Why are there so few treatments for Alzheimer's?

The blood–brain barrier was originally discovered by German doctor Paul Ehrlich when he injected dye into the bloodstream of a mouse. He was surprised when the dye was carried throughout the animal's body but did not enter the brain and spinal cord. Ehrlich hypothesized that an invisible barrier must exist in the body to protect the central nervous system.

Later, in the 1960s, scientists were able to use powerful microscopes to examine the blood–brain barrier in detail. They found that endothelial cells lined the blood vessels with tight junctions in between each cell. The blood–brain barrier is very effective at keeping unwanted pathogens out of the brain. Unfortunately, this barrier is also effective against Alzheimer's drugs and therapies.

Scientists are currently trying to devise ways of breaching the blood–brain barrier for beneficial drugs. In one method, called the "Trojan horse approach," a drug is fused to a molecule that can pass through the blood–brain barrier safely. Another option is using ultrasound to temporarily open the blood–brain barrier to let in medicine. Both methods are currently being studied and will hopefully lead to new treatment options in the future.

Yoga for Alzheimer's disease

There have been a few studies published on how yoga-related practices impact people with mild cognitive impairment, dementia and cognitive decline (Brenes *et al.*, 2019; Bhattacharyya, Andel and Small, 2021). Researchers at Wake Forest School of Medicine reviewed 12 studies examining the impact of yoga on people with mild cognitive impairment and dementia (Brenes *et al.*, 2019). They found across the studies that practicing yoga helped to improve cognitive functioning, sleep, mood and, possibly, neural connectivity.

Improved cognitive functioning included memory and attention, which can both be severely affected in mild cognitive impairment and dementia. Sleep disorders are also common, and disturbances in sleep may affect cognitive functioning, as memory consolidation largely takes place during sleep. Yoga has been shown to improve sleep quality as well as the number of hours of sleep. Thus, yoga may act as a mediator for improving cognitive functioning through improved sleep (Brenes *et al.*, 2019).

Mood disorders, such as anxiety and depression, often occur with mild cognitive impairment and dementia. Five of the studies reviewed found improvements in symptoms of anxiety and depression after the yoga intervention. A decrease in psychiatric symptoms could potentially lead to less caregiver burnout, the authors point out (Brenes *et al.*, 2019). While the studies used a variety of styles of yoga and different intervention protocols, yoga appears to be a safe and beneficial tool for improving health in those with mild cognitive impairment and dementia.

Another recent review conducted by researchers from the School of Aging Studies at the University of South Florida analyzed 11 randomized control trials that investigated the effects of yoga-related mind–body therapies on cognitive function, in the context of aging (Bhattacharyya, Andel and Small, 2021). Over 900 participants were included in the studies. No adverse effects were reported in any of the studies, and the results revealed that yoga-related therapies improved memory, executive function, attention and processing speed in older adults with and without cognitive impairment.

These review articles provide preliminary evidence that yoga could be an effective method for improving health in those with mild cognitive impairment, dementia and cognitive decline. Future studies need to be conducted to see if these results hold true in those specifically with Alzheimer's.

Meditation may also offer benefits through decreasing stress and inflammation. High levels of the stress hormone cortisol can damage the brain's memory center, the hippocampus. Decreasing stress could reduce the amount of cumulative damage to the hippocampus and, possibly, slow down or halt memory degradation, a hallmark of Alzheimer's. One small study of 14 participants found a trend towards less hippocampal cell death in the mindfulness-based stress reduction group compared with the control group (Wells *et al.*, 2013).

Although there are only a few studies on the effects of yoga and meditation on mild cognitive impairment and dementia, they do seem to suggest there is some benefit. Yoga and meditation practices are both safe and feasible in the older adult population. Larger, more rigorous studies still need to be completed to better understand the full effects.

> **Main takeaways**
> - **Alzheimer's disease** is an eventually fatal dementia with no effective treatment options.
> - The **blood–brain barrier** is a filter between the brain's blood vessels and the brain tissue.
> - The two main biomarkers associated with Alzheimer's are amyloid beta plaques and tau proteins.
> - Genetics, diet, exercise, education and breach of the blood–brain barrier may also impact the development of Alzheimer's.
> - Yoga may improve memory, attention, sleep, mood, anxiety and depression.
> - Meditation could decrease damage in the hippocampus by lowering overall stress, which reduces the stress hormone cortisol.

PAIN AND THE BRAIN

Pain can be acute, stemming from an immediate cause, or chronic, spanning weeks, years or even a lifetime. Pain is complex and does not originate from a single region of the brain. Instead, it involves multiple areas that work together to process signals. Pain has physical and emotional components; physical pain can be the cause of psychological and emotional stress, but it can also be the result.

Physical pain uses specialized pain-sensing neurons called **nociceptors**. Nociceptors detect tissue-damaging stimuli in either the skin or internal organs, for example, the bladder or the digestive tract (Blumenrath, 2020). Normal touch does not trigger a nociceptor but tripping and falling will. Different nociceptors detect distinct types of pain, such as thermal pain (too hot or too cold), physical pain (wound) or chemical pain (toxin). Nociceptors send messages about pain to the brain using different pathways, depending on the type of pain experienced.

Nociceptors rely on nerves called A-delta and C-fibers to transmit information. The A-delta fibers are myelinated (just like neurons), so that pain signals travel quickly to the brain; whereas C-fibers are not myelinated, and messages travel more slowly. A-delta fibers are useful for communicating sharp and sudden pain, while C-fibers relay information about dull, aching pain.

Pain signals travel to the spinal cord, which in turn passes the information on to the thalamus in the brain. The thalamus is the relay center and sends the message to the cerebral cortex to generate the experience and awareness of the pain. Although the brain is an advanced organ, it cannot always accurately pinpoint the origin of pain in the body. A person experiencing a heart attack may feel "referred pain" in the left arm. Scientists are not exactly sure why this occurs, but it may be because some of the pain fibers overlap in the spinal cord, leading to crossed wiring.

The brain is influenced by things like attention, mood and emotional state when processing the experience of pain (Bushnell, Čeko and Low, 2013). For example, bringing attention to a wound can make the pain feel worse. If attention is redirected, the feelings of pain can be reduced. This redirection of attention and reduction of pain can be harnessed using mindfulness meditation.

Emotional pain is as real as physical pain. In fact, common pain relievers such as acetaminophen relieve emotional pain (Mischkowski, Crocker and Way, 2019). The regulation of the emotional aspect of pain is thought to depend on an area in the brainstem called the periaqueductal gray matter. This brain region increases or decreases feelings of pain depending on emotional state. For example, feeling empathetic about a friend's pain can increase our own feelings of pain (Bushnell, Čeko and Low, 2013). Emotional pain has also been shown to activate many of the same brain regions as physical pain (Kross et al., 2011).

Not all messages about pain travel to the brain. Accidentally touching a hot pan will initiate the reflex of pulling the hand back. This action is so fast that it is processed without the brain. Instead, sensory neurons send signals from the hand to the spinal cord, where the information is passed on to a motor neuron that sends signals back to the hand to initiate movement.

> **Main takeaways**
> - Pain can be both a physical and emotional experience.
> - **Nociceptors** detect thermal, physical and chemical pain.
> - Fast, myelinated A-delta fibers transmit signals about sharp pain, while slow, unmyelinated C-fibers send signals about dull, aching pain.
> - Feeling pain is influenced by attention, mood and emotional state.
> - Mindfulness meditation can reduce feelings of pain by redirecting attention.

CHRONIC PAIN

It is estimated that approximately 20 percent of American adults experience chronic pain (Dahlhamer et al., 2018). **Chronic pain** is pain that lasts more than three months, and it can affect relationships, quality of life and productivity (American Society of Anesthesiologists, 2021).

Although we do not fully understand the origins of chronic pain, scientists have observed brain changes in regions associated with emotion, attention and pain regulation (Bushnell, Čeko and Low, 2013). These brain changes may cause the perception of pain to be enhanced, leading to an overactive nervous system.

Chronic pain can persist even when an injury has healed. For example, complex regional pain syndrome (CRPS) is a form of chronic pain that usually affects an arm or leg after an injury. While poorly understood and with limited treatment options, CRPS typically occurs after physical trauma, such as a broken bone. The chronic pain can be so debilitating that nearly 50 percent of individuals with CRPS contemplate suicide (Sharma et al., 2009). The intense pain is thought to be due to nerve damage that occurred during the injury. The brain becomes confused and thinks the injury is still occurring, even after it has healed. It may also be due to an overactive sympathetic nervous system, but more research needs to be conducted.

Successful treatments for chronic pain, aside from medications, often focus on the emotional component of pain involving the brain's limbic system. Contemplative practices, like meditation, can alter the emotional and attentional pain pathways to reduce pain (Bushnell, Čeko and Low, 2013). Researchers from Ben Gurion University of the Negev in Israel reviewed 16 studies on the effect of mindfulness on chronic pain, half of which were controlled studies (Strauss et al., 2014). Six of the eight controlled trials showed that mindfulness-based interventions could successfully reduce pain intensity.

In a more extensive review of 38 studies, researchers looked at the use of mindfulness meditation for chronic pain and found that there was a small decrease in pain and symptoms of depression with an overall improvement in quality of life (Hilton et al., 2016). Despite the overall quality of the studies being low, there does seem to be some level of pain reduction for those who practice meditation.

Main takeaways
- **Chronic pain** is pain that lasts more than three months, and it can affect relationships, quality of life and productivity.
- Chronic pain involves changes in brain regions involved in emotion, attention and pain regulation.
- Meditation can alter the emotional and attentional pain pathways to reduce pain.

Mindfulness meditation for reducing pain
Come into a comfortable position and start to notice the sounds around you. Bring awareness to the sounds from inside as well as any sounds from outside. Bring in any sounds from nature into your field of perception. Focus on the harmony of all of the sounds together. Bring awareness to the air that is bringing these sounds to your ears. Feel the air around your body. Notice the air that comes in and out of the body through breathing. Bring focus to this air. In and out. Can you feel the sensations of the breath coming in and out? How does the breath affect your whole body? Feel the ribs expand as air comes in. Feel the abs tighten as the air is pushed out. Notice how the whole body acts together to breathe. Start to bring attention to one region of your body that is not hurting. Focus on the sensations in that region. Now bring awareness to a part of your body that is hurting. Turn towards the pain and the intensity of the sensations. For a few seconds, observe this feeling with a hint of openness. Now reflect on that moment. How did it feel? How is it in this new moment after allowing the pain to be in the body? Although that openness was quick, it is the start of developing a new relationship with the way you feel pain.

Lower back pain

Lower back pain is one of the most common and debilitating types of chronic pain. The American College of Physicians currently recommends yoga and mindfulness-based stress reduction as a non-drug therapy option for treatment (Qaseem et al., 2017). A growing body of evidence suggests that contemplative practices are effective at promoting back health by redirecting attention and improving physical functioning. Researchers from the University of Maryland reviewed 12 studies with 1,080 participants and found that practicing yoga (mostly Iyengar, Hatha or Viniyoga) resulted in small to moderate improvements in back-related function after three and six months of active practice (Wieland et al., 2017). In another study, researchers from the University of York in the UK conducted a large, randomized trial of yoga for chronic lower back pain (Tilbrook et al., 2011). They looked at the effect of a three-month yoga program on lower back function and pain over a year in comparison with a control group. Their results showed that the yoga group had better back function and reported less pain at three and six months compared with the group that received usual care.

Chronic back pain affects many veterans, and researchers from the University of California, San

Diego examined the benefits of yoga on 150 military veterans (Groessl *et al.*, 2017). Yoga classes were offered twice a week for three months and consisted of physical postures, movement and breathing techniques. The researchers found that pain intensity improved after three and six months, although the decrease in pain intensity was small.

Meditation is another effective treatment option for people experiencing lower back pain. Scientists at the University of Washington conducted a rigorous, randomized clinical trial examining the differences between cognitive behavioral therapy, usual care and mindfulness-based stress reduction in adults with chronic lower back pain (Cherkin, Sherman and Balderson, 2016). Cognitive behavioral therapy involves changing pain-related thoughts and behaviors. Mindfulness-based stress reduction is an intensive mindfulness training that teaches the practitioner to think about pain with curiosity and openness to change their perception of pain.

The well-designed study included 342 adults between the ages of 20 and 70 years old. Participants were randomly assigned to a condition, and the interviewer was not aware of the group assignments of the participants. At the six-month mark, participants in the cognitive behavioral therapy and meditation groups showed more improvement in levels of back pain than the usual care group, which included any care participants received outside of the intervention. These results held strong after a year, with no major differences between the cognitive behavioral therapy and meditation groups. The results of this study suggest that both cognitive behavioral therapy and meditation may offer a treatment advantage over usual care for chronic lower back pain. Overall, mindfulness meditation should be considered as a line of treatment for individuals experiencing lower back pain.

Main takeaways
- Yoga and meditation are recommended for the treatment of lower back pain.
- Yoga can improve back function and reduce pain intensity.
- Meditation is more effective than usual care at reducing back pain.

EXAMPLE NEUTRAL SPINE YOGA FLOW

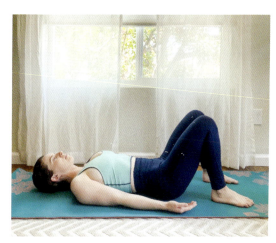

Figure 9.20 Corpse pose variation with bent legs to reduce strain on lower back.

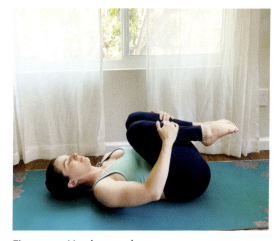

Figure 9.21 Hug legs to chest.

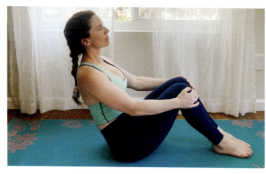

Figure 9.22 Supported boat pose.

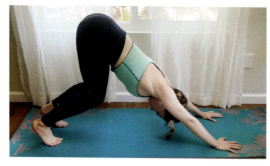

Figure 9.23 Downward-facing dog variation with bent knees.

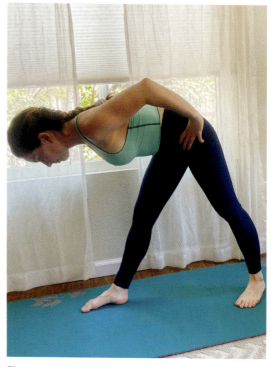

Figure 9.25 Triangle pose variation.

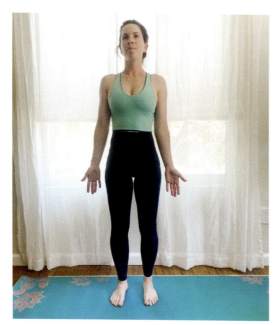

Figure 9.24 Mountain pose with slight bend in the knees.

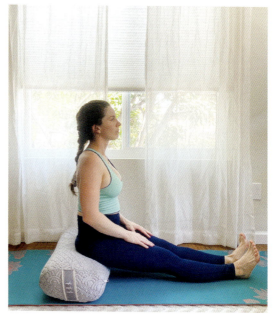

Figure 9.26 Supported seated pose with bolster to align the spine.

ARTHRITIS

Arthritis affects millions of people in the United States every year. About one in four adults with arthritis report experiencing severe joint pain, according to the Centers for Disease Control and Prevention (CDC, 2022b). In addition, nearly half of adults with arthritis have persistent pain. The two main forms of arthritis are rheumatoid arthritis and osteoarthritis, and both forms of the disease can lead to chronic pain.

Rheumatoid arthritis is a chronic inflammatory disorder affecting the joints. It occurs when the body's immune system attacks the body's own tissues. The resulting inflammation can damage other parts of the body as well, impacting quality of life (Evans et al., 2013).

Yoga can improve quality of life and health for those with rheumatoid arthritis. Researchers from the University of California, Los Angeles conducted a study looking at a twice-a-week Iyengar yoga program on measures of health in individuals with rheumatoid arthritis (Evans et al., 2013). The six-week intervention included 11 participants and 15 controls who completed usual care, which consisted of the routine care participants received for rheumatoid arthritis. The individuals who completed the yoga training showed significantly greater improvement in quality of life, pain, mood, fatigue and general health in comparison with the control group. Notably, almost half of the yoga group reported clinically relevant improvement in their arthritis symptoms. These improvements were still evident at the two-month follow-up. Thus, yoga appears to be an effective complementary treatment for rheumatoid arthritis.

In addition to yoga, a review conducted by researchers at Harvard Medical School found that meditation-based interventions were largely effective at improving symptoms of rheumatoid arthritis (Koulouris et al., 2018). Across nine randomized control trials and four other studies, meditation was found to decrease pain, inflammation and fatigue, as well as a number of other measures.

Osteoarthritis occurs when the cartilage between bones breaks down, damaging the joints. Eventually, the cartilage can wear down to such an extent that bone can rub on bone, causing even more damage. Currently, the American College of Rheumatology and the Arthritis Foundation recommend yoga as a treatment for the management of osteoarthritis of the hand, hip and knee (Kolasinski et al., 2020). Yoga may help to improve mobility of the joints, making the joints feel less stiff.

Scientists from the University of Technology Sydney in Australia reviewed nine randomized control trials to better understand the effect of yoga on osteoarthritis (Lauche et al., 2019). The studies included 640 individuals, largely with osteoarthritis of the lower limb (mainly the knee). The analysis showed that yoga was effective for improving pain, function and stiffness in osteoarthritis of the knee. However, the authors do note that many of the studies were low quality (Lauche et al., 2019).

There have not been many studies conducted on the benefit of meditation for those with osteoarthritis. In one study, scientists from West Virginia University conducted a randomized clinical trial examining the effects of mantra meditation in comparison with listening to music on knee pain in older adults with osteoarthritis (Innes et al., 2018). Twenty-two adults were split between the meditation group and the music listening group, and they were asked to practice 15–20 minutes twice daily for eight weeks. Both groups demonstrated improvements in knee pain, function, mood, stress and overall health. When comparing the groups with one another, the meditation group showed larger improvements in mood, sleep and mental health than the music listening group. Thus, mantra meditation, and possibly listening to music, may be a complementary treatment for osteoarthritis.

> **Main takeaways**
> - Rheumatoid arthritis is a chronic inflammatory disorder affecting the joints. Yoga can improve quality of life, pain, mood and fatigue.
> - Osteoarthritis occurs when the cartilage between bones breaks down, damaging the joints. Yoga may help to improve mobility of joints, pain, function and stiffness for those with osteoarthritis of the knee. Mantra meditation may also benefit those with osteoarthritis, although studies are inconclusive.

YOGA EXERCISES FOR INDIVIDUALS WITH ARTHRITIS

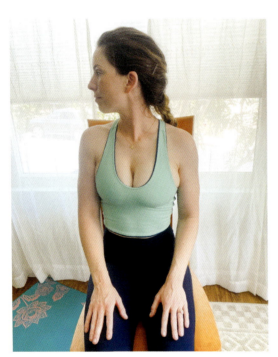

Figure 9.27 Look left and right to stretch the neck.

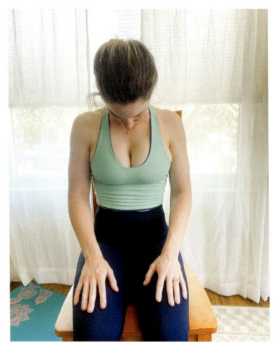

Figure 9.28 Look up and down, paying attention not to extend too far in either direction.

THE EFFECT OF YOGA AND MEDITATION ON THE BRAIN

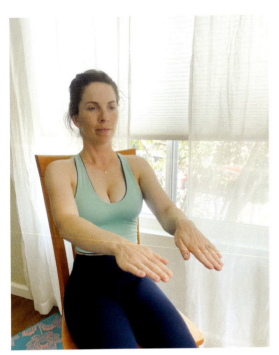

Figure 9.29 Raise arms in front and close the fingers.

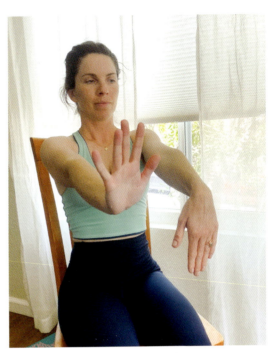

Figure 9.31 Move the hands up and down to flex the wrists.

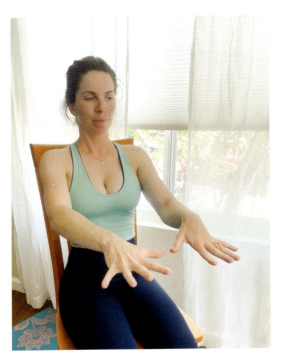

Figure 9.30 Spread the fingers.

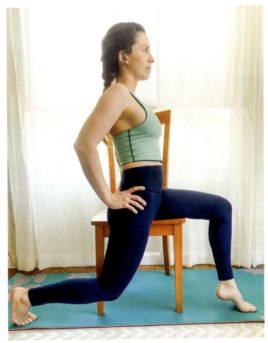

Figure 9.32 Chair-assisted forward lunge.

ADDICTION

Treatment-induced addiction

Patients with chronic pain are often prescribed powerfully addictive drugs, such as opioids, that activate the reward centers in the brain. Pain-related anxiety also appears to be related to tobacco dependence among those with chronic pain (Ditre et al., 2013).

Addiction is a treatable, chronic medical disease involving complex interactions among brain circuits, genetics, the environment and an individual's life, according to the American Society of Addiction Medicine (ASAM, 2022). People with addiction will use drugs even when they know their use will cause harm or other problems.

Addiction is associated with alterations in mood, personality and behavioral changes as well as structural and functional brain changes (Kosten and George, 2002). Some of the more common brain regions implicated in addiction are the prefrontal cortex, the amygdala and the basal ganglia, key regions of the brain's reward network.

To recap from previous chapters, the prefrontal cortex is the brain's control center. This large region encompassing the front of the brain is important for making decisions, solving problems and exerting self-control. The amygdala is the brain's fear center and plays a role in experiencing the anxiety and unease that occurs when coming off an addictive drug. This region can become increasingly sensitive with continued drug use. Lastly, the basal ganglia are part of the brain's motivation center and help process pleasure; this group of neurons is also involved in the formation of habits and routines, both good and bad.

Some drugs affect more than just the reward-processing regions of the brain. Drugs such as opioids also target the brainstem, which is responsible for basic functions like breathing. Opioids have been shown to bind to receptors in a specific group of neurons in the brainstem that are responsible for maintaining breathing. Once the drugs bind, these neurons cause disrupted breathing, and ultimately respiratory arrest, causing overdose deaths (Liu et al., 2021).

Many drugs interfere with the way neurons send and receive information. For example, the nicotine in tobacco crosses the blood–brain barrier and binds to receptors in the brain, tricking the brain into becoming more active and releasing more neurotransmitters like dopamine and acetylcholine. While an increase in dopamine strengthens the experience of pleasure, an increase in acetylcholine could be the cause of increased attention and cognition observed after smoking cigarettes. After multiple uses, the brain gets used to a certain level of stimulation, called tolerance. Thus, the person will need to inhale more and more nicotine to experience the same positive effects. Tolerance is different to dependency, which is due to physiological demands or psychological feelings that a person cannot function properly without using a substance.

Yoga has been shown to be helpful in treating multiple types of addictions, including alcohol, drug and nicotine addiction (Walia et al., 2021). In a review of eight randomized control trials, researchers from Liverpool John Moores University and the University of Exeter in the UK found that yoga can reduce stress and addictive behaviors while also improving self-esteem and self-control (Posadzki et al., 2014). Although many of the studies reviewed were low quality, the results are encouraging that yoga may be a beneficial tool for treating addiction.

Nicotine addiction

Using contemplative practices to treat nicotine addiction has been heavily studied, and the results show that meditation, and possibly yoga, can reduce cigarette use.

Nicotine is the addictive component in tobacco, and there are an estimated 1.3 billion tobacco users worldwide (World Health Organization, 2021). Despite the popularity and prevalence, cigarette smoking is the leading cause of preventable disease, disability and death in the United States, and the leading cause of preventable death globally (Brewer et al., 2011). Studies show that many smokers want to stop smoking but feel unable to do so.

Stress is a major trigger for smoking cigarettes. When the brain experiences stress, the prefrontal cortex stops functioning properly. Mindfulness meditation can be useful for connecting the smoker with their own experience. This can help to lower stress levels and alleviate the feelings of needing to smoke. Learning to be more mindful of one's experiences can also help smokers become more aware of their feelings and understand the reasons why they are reaching for a cigarette in the first place. Meditation also helps boost self-control, which is a critical aspect of overcoming any addiction.

Neuroscientist and addiction psychiatrist Judson Brewer, author of *The Craving Mind*, is a leader in examining how mindfulness meditation can impact addiction, particularly to nicotine. Brewer breaks down nicotine addiction (or any harmful habit) into three main steps: 1) trigger, 2) behavior, and 3) reward. For example, you can be feeling sad (trigger), so you grab some ice cream from the freezer (behavior) and then you start to feel better (reward). It works the same with nicotine. You might feel stressed (trigger), reach for a cigarette (behavior) and then feel some relief (reward). Each time this process occurs the brain is being trained and circuits are being rewired, eventually leading to the formation of a habit.

Brewer's research group has conducted multiple studies to examine if mindfulness can help people quit smoking. In the studies, the researchers prompt the participants to cultivate curiosity. They allow the participants to keep smoking as long as the smokers concentrate on what it truly feels like to smoke a cigarette. Brewer has found that when people bring attention to the smell and taste of tobacco, smoking becomes much less desirable (Brewer, 2016).

In one seminal study, Brewer's research group found that mindfulness training was twice as effective as the gold standard therapy for smoking cessation. The rigorous, randomized clinical control trial consisted of 88 nicotine-dependent adults (Brewer et al., 2011). The scientists were interested to see if mindfulness could be as beneficial as the American Lung Association's Freedom from Smoking treatment. Participants were randomly assigned to each group, and treatments were delivered twice a week for one month.

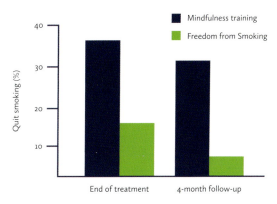

Figure 9.33 Individuals who completed the mindfulness training were more likely to quit smoking than the Freedom from Smoking control group.

Participants smoked an average of 20 cigarettes a day at the start of the study. Individuals who completed the mindfulness training showed a greater reduction in cigarette use during the treatment and at the four-month follow-up visit than the Freedom from Smoking treatment group (Figure 9.33). This was a well-designed, rigorous study, and the results suggest that mindfulness training may be even more effective at smoking cessation than the current standard treatments, such as Freedom from Smoking (Brewer et al., 2011).

Yoga for nicotine addiction has also been studied, although with less conclusive results. In a large clinical trial of 227 participants, researchers from Brown University examined if yoga could be an effective aid for smoking cessation (Bock et al., 2018). Participants in the study smoked an average of 17 cigarettes a day and were randomly assigned to an eight-week program of Iyengar yoga (twice weekly) or general wellness classes as a control. All participants underwent a cognitive-behavioral smoking cessation program as well. Follow-ups were conducted at eight weeks, three months and six months.

Results showed that the yoga group had a 37 percent higher likelihood of quitting smoking than the general wellness group. The scientists also observed a dose effect in the yoga group, meaning that each additional yoga class attended increased the participants' likelihood of quitting smoking by roughly 12 percent (Bock et al., 2018).

Main takeaways

- **Addiction** is a treatable, chronic medical disease involving complex interactions among brain circuits, genetics, the environment and an individual's life experiences.
- Yoga can reduce stress and addictive behaviors while also improving self-esteem and self-control.
- Yoga and meditation are effective alternative options for treating nicotine addiction.
- Mindfulness meditation practice can help to rewire the brain to reduce stress and cravings.

REFERENCES

American Association of Neurological Surgeons (AANS), 2020. Traumatic brain injury. Available at: https://www.aans.org/Patients/Neurosurgical-Conditions-and-Treatments/Traumatic-Brain-Injury#:~:text=An%20estimated%2013.5%20million%20individuals,hospitalizations%20for%20spinal%20cord%20injury

American Society of Anesthesiologists, 2021. Chronic pain. Available at: https://www.asahq.org/madeforthismoment/pain-management/types-of-pain/chronic/#:~:text=Chronic%20pain%20is%20pain%20that,lasting%20three%20months%20or%20longer

Acabchuk, R.L., Brisson, J.M., Park, C.L., Babbott-Bryan, N., Parmelee, O.A., & Johnson, B.T., 2020. Therapeutic effects of meditation, yoga, and mindfulness-based interventions for chronic symptoms of mild traumatic brain injury: a systematic review and meta-analysis. *Applied Psychology: Health and Well-Being*, 13(1), pp.34–62.

American Society of Addiction Medicine (ASAM), 2022. Definition of addiction. Available at: www.asam.org/quality-care/definition-of-addiction

Ates, G., Goldberg, J., Currais, A., & Maher, P., 2020. CMS121, a fatty acid synthase inhibitor, protects against excess lipid peroxidation and inflammation and alleviates cognitive loss in a transgenic mouse model of Alzheimer's disease. *Redox Biology*, 36, p.101648.

Bhattacharyya, K. K., Andel, R., & Small, B.J. 2021. Effects of yoga-related mind–body therapies on cognitive function in older adults: a systematic review with meta-analysis. *Archives of Gerontology and Geriatrics*, 93, Article 104319.

Blumenrath, S., 2020. The neuroscience of touch and pain. Available at: https://www.brainfacts.org/thinking-sensing-and-behaving/touch/2020/the-neuroscience-of-touch-and-pain-013020

Bock, B.C., Dunsiger, S.I., Rosen, R.K., Thind, H., et al., 2018. Yoga as a complementary therapy for smoking cessation: results from BreathEasy, a randomized clinical trial. *Nicotine & Tobacco Research*, 21(11), pp.1517–1523.

Brenes, G.A., Sohl, S., Wells, R.E., Befus, D., Campos, C.L., & Danhauer, S.C., 2019. The effects of yoga on patients with mild cognitive impairment and dementia: a scoping review. *The American Journal of Geriatric Psychiatry*, 27(2), pp.188–197.

Brewer, J., 2016. *A simple way to break a bad habit*, TED Talks. Available at: https://www.youtube.com/watch?v=-moW9jvvMr4

Brewer, J.A., Mallik, S., Babuscio, T.A., Nich, C., et al., 2011. Mindfulness training for smoking cessation: results from a randomized controlled trial. *Drug and Alcohol Dependence*, 119(1–2), pp.72–80.

Bushnell, M.C., Čeko, M., & Low, L.A., 2013. Cognitive and emotional control of pain and its disruption in chronic pain. *Nature Reviews Neuroscience*, 14(7), pp.502–511.

Cavalera, C., Rovaris, M., Mendozzi, L., Pugnetti, L., et al., 2018. Online meditation training for people with multiple sclerosis: a randomized controlled trial. *Multiple Sclerosis Journal*, 25(4), pp.610–617.

Centers for Disease Control and Prevention (CDC), 2022a. Stroke facts. Available at: www.cdc.gov/stroke/facts.htm

Centers for Disease Control and Prevention (CDC), 2022b. Joint pain. Available at: www.cdc.gov/arthritis/pain

Cherkin, D.C., Sherman, K.J., & Balderson, B.H., 2016. Effect of mindfulness-based stress reduction vs cognitive behavioral therapy or usual care on back pain and functional limitations in adults with chronic low back pain. *JAMA*, 315(12), p.1240.

Dahlhamer, J., Lucas, J., Zelaya, C., Nahin, R., et al., 2018. Prevalence of chronic pain and high-impact chronic pain among adults — United States, 2016. *Morbidity and Mortality Weekly Report*, 67(36), pp.1001-1006.

Ditre, J.W., Zale, E.L., Kosiba, J.D., & Zvolensky, M.J., 2013. A pilot study of pain-related anxiety and smoking dependence motives among persons with chronic pain. *Experimental Clinical Psychopharmacololgy*, 21(6), pp.443-449.

Donnelly, K.Z., Baker, K., Pierce, R., St. Ivany, A.R., Barr, P.J., & Bruce, M.L., 2019. A retrospective study on the acceptability, feasibility, and effectiveness of LoveYourBrain Yoga for people with traumatic brain injury and caregivers. *Disability and Rehabilitation*, 43(12), pp.1764-1775.

Donnelly, K.Z., Goldberg, S., & Fournier, D., 2019. A qualitative study of LoveYourBrain Yoga: a group-based yoga with psychoeducation intervention to facilitate community integration for people with traumatic brain injury and their caregivers. *Disability and Rehabilitation*, 42(17), pp.2482-2491.

Evans, S., Moieni, M., Lung, K., Tsao, J., et al., 2013. Impact of Iyengar yoga on quality of life in young women with rheumatoid arthritis. *The Clinical Journal of Pain*, 29(11), pp.988-997.

Friedman, A., Kaufer, D., Shemer, J., Hendler, I., Soreq, H., & Tur-Kaspa, I. 1996. Pyridostigmine brain penetration under stress enhances neuronal excitability and induces early immediate transcriptional response. *Nature Medicine*, 2(12), pp.1382-1385.

Garrett, R., Immink, M.A., & Hillier, S., 2011. Becoming connected: the lived experience of yoga participation after stroke. *Disability and Rehabilitation*, 33(25-26), pp.2404-2415.

Groessl, E.J., Liu, L., Chang, D.G., Wetherell, J.L., et al., 2017. Yoga for military veterans with chronic low back pain: a randomized clinical trial. *American Journal of Preventive Medicine*, 53(5), pp.599-608.

Hilton, L., Hempel, S., Ewing, B.A., Apaydin, E., et al., 2016. Mindfulness meditation for chronic pain: systematic review and meta-analysis. *Annals of Behavioral Medicine*, 51(2), pp.199-213.

Innes, K.E., Selfe, T.K., Kandati, S., Wen, S., & Huysmans, Z., 2018. Effects of mantra meditation versus music listening on knee pain, function, and related outcomes in older adults with knee osteoarthritis: an exploratory randomized clinical trial (RCT). *Evidence-Based Complementary and Alternative Medicine*, 2018, pp.1-19.

Johns Hopkins Medicine, 2022. Traumatic brain injury. Available at: https://www.hopkinsmedicine.org/health/conditions-and-diseases/traumatic-brain-injury

Kolasinski, S.L., Neogi, T., Hochberg, M.C., Oatis, C., et al., 2020. 2019 American College of Rheumatology/Arthritis Foundation guideline for the management of osteoarthritis of the hand, hip, and knee. *Arthritis & Rheumatology*, 72(2), pp.220-233.

Kosten, T., & George, T., 2002. The neurobiology of opioid dependence: implications for treatment. *Science & Practice Perspectives*, 1(1), pp.13-20.

Koulouris, A., Dorado, K., McDonnell, C., Edwards, R.R., & Lazaridou, A., 2018. A review of the efficacy of yoga and meditation-based interventions for rheumatoid arthritis. *OBM Integrative and Complementary Medicine*, 3(3).

Kross, E., Berman, M.G., Mischel, W., Smith, E.E., & Wager, T.D., 2011. Social rejection shares somatosensory representations with physical pain. *Proceedings of the National Academy of Sciences*, 108(15), pp.6270-6275.

Kunkle, B.W., Grenier-Boley, B., Sims, R., Bis, J.C., et al., 2019. Genetic meta-analysis of diagnosed Alzheimer's disease identifies new risk loci and implicates AB, Tau, immunity and lipid processing. *Nature Genetics*, 51(3), pp.414-430.

Larkin, M., 2000. Meditation may reduce heart attack and stroke risk. *The Lancet*, 355(9206), p.812.

Lauche, R., Hunter, D.J., Adams, J., & Cramer, H., 2019. Yoga for osteoarthritis: a systematic review and meta-analysis. *Current Rheumatology Reports*, 21(9), p.47.

Lawrence, M., Celestino Jr., F.T., Matozinho, H.H.S., Govan, L., Booth, J., & Beecher, J., 2017. Yoga for stroke rehabilitation. *Cochrane Database of Systematic Reviews*, 2017(12), CD011483.

Levin, A.B., Hadgkiss, E.J., Weiland, T.J., Jelinek, G.A., et al., 2014. Meditation as an adjunct to the management of multiple sclerosis. *Neurology Research International*, 2014, pp.1-10.

Liu, S., Kim, D.-I., Oh, T.G., & Pao, G.M., 2021. Neural basis of opioid-induced respiratory depression and its rescue. *Proceedings of the National Academy of Sciences*, 118(23), e2022134118.

Minvaleev, R.S., Bogdanov, R.R., Bahner, D.P., & Levitov, A.B., 2019. Headstand (Sirshasana) does not increase the blood flow to the brain. *The Journal of Alternative and Complementary Medicine*, 25(8), pp.827-832.

Mischkowski, D., Crocker, J., & Way, B.M., 2019. A social analgesic? Acetaminophen (paracetamol) reduces positive empathy. *Frontiers in Psychology*, 10, p.538.

National Multiple Sclerosis Society, 2022. Types of MS. Available at: https://www.nationalmssociety.org/What-is-MS/Types-of-MS

Posadzki, P., Choi, J., Lee, M.S., & Ernst, E., 2014. Yoga for addictions: a systematic review of randomised clinical trials. *Focus on Alternative and Complementary Therapies*, 19(1), pp.1-8.

Qaseem, A., Wilt, T.J., McLean, R.M., & Forciea, M.A., 2017. Noninvasive treatments for acute, subacute, and chronic low back pain: a clinical practice guideline from the American College of Physicians. *Annals of Internal Medicine*, 166(7), p.514.

Senatorov, V.V., Friedman, A.R., Milikovsky, D.Z., Ofer, J., et al., 2019. Blood–brain barrier dysfunction in aging induces hyperactivation of TGFB signaling and chronic yet reversible neural dysfunction. *Science Translational Medicine*, 11(521), eaaw8283.

Sharma, A., Agarwal, S., Broatch, J., & Raja, S.N., 2009. A web-based cross-sectional epidemiological survey of complex regional pain syndrome. *Regional Anesthesia and Pain Medicine*, 34(2), pp.110–115.

Strauss, C., Cavanagh, K., Oliver, A., & Pettman, D., 2014. Mindfulness-based interventions for people diagnosed with a current episode of an anxiety or depressive disorder: a meta-analysis of randomised controlled trials. *PLoS ONE*, 9(4), e96110.

Stump, E., 2009. How Natasha Richardson's death put brain injury in the spotlight. Available at: https://www.brainandlife.org/articles/the-tragic-death-of-natasha-richardson

Thayabaranathan, T., Andrew, N.E., Immink, M.A., Hillier, S., *et al.*, 2017. Determining the potential benefits of yoga in chronic stroke care: a systematic review and meta-analysis. *Topics in Stroke Rehabilitation*, 24(4), pp.279–287.

Tilbrook, H.E., Cox, H., Hewitt, C.E., Kang'ombe, A.R., *et al.*, 2011. Yoga for chronic low back pain. *Annals of Internal Medicine*, 155(9), p.569.

Walia, N., Matas, J., Turner, A., Gonzalez, S., & Zoorob, R., 2021. Yoga for substance use: a systematic review. *The Journal of the American Board of Family Medicine*, 34(5), pp.964–973.

Wathugala, M., Saldana, D., Juliano, J.M., Chan, J., & Liew, S.-L., 2019. Mindfulness meditation effects on poststroke spasticity: a feasibility study. *Journal of Evidence-Based Integrative Medicine*, 24, 2515690X19855941.

Wells, R.E., Yeh, G.Y., Kerr, C.E., Wolkin, J., *et al.*, 2013. Meditation's impact on default mode network and hippocampus in mild cognitive impairment: a pilot study. *Neuroscience Letters*, 556, pp.15–19.

Wieland, L.S., Skoetz, N., Pilkington, K., Vempati, R., D'Adamo, C.R., & Berman, B.M., 2017. Yoga treatment for chronic non-specific low back pain. *Cochrane Database of Systematic Reviews*, 2017(1), CD010671.

World Health Organization, 2021. Tobacco. Available at: https://www.who.int/news-room/fact-sheets/detail/tobacco

CHAPTER 10

Healthy Aging, Yoga and the Brain

The brain changes throughout the lifespan. Our experiences, both internal and external, help shape us into the person we are. Practicing yoga and meditation can be beneficial at any age – infancy, childhood, adolescence, adulthood and old age. This chapter will explore the science behind how these practices may improve brain health, promote well-being and slow the aging process to improve quality of life and add years of healthy living.

THE EARLY YEARS: INFANCY AND EARLY CHILDHOOD

The human brain experiences extraordinary changes throughout gestation, infancy and early childhood. At birth, a baby's brain is a quarter of the size of an adult's brain (Ikeda and Teasdale, 2018). Although white matter tracts are established before birth, these axons become myelinated during the first two years of life. The myelination allows for faster neuron-to-neuron communication. Gray matter also expands rapidly during this period, and the thickness of the cortex peaks between one and two years (Gilmore, Knickmeyer and Gao, 2018). By two years of age, the young brain has grown to three quarters the size of an adult brain (Ikeda and Teasdale, 2018).

During the first few years of life, more than 1 million new connections are created between neurons every second (Harvard University, 2007). The infant brain is considered plastic and malleable, so it is easy to influence developing brain architecture. The first brain pathways to develop are those involving the senses such as vision and hearing. Next, the language circuits start to develop, followed by more complex, higher cognitive function. Unused connections are reduced or pruned back so that brain circuits can become more efficient.

Brain development is influenced by both genes and experiences. While genes provide a blueprint, experiences influence which genes are expressed. For example, young children seek affirmation, kindness and affection from caregivers. Nurturing care is fundamental for a thriving brain. If the infant or child does not receive such responses or experiences, structures in their brain may be altered, making them more susceptible to learning and behavioral differences. The early years build the foundation for future brain health.

Yoga for young minds

The young brain is impressionable and built for learning. Infancy and young childhood are wonderful times to introduce contemplative practices to stimulate brain development and promote emotional and physical learning. Infant or baby yoga typically consists of gentle stretches and movements to music for infants starting at three months old. These slow, controlled movements help with muscle and nerve development. Certain movements like bicycle legs may aid the baby's digestive system by relieving built-up gas, while positions on the tummy help to build upper back and neck muscles (MacDonald, 2013). Infant yoga may also improve sleep patterns and reduce levels of stress hormones, such as cortisol, although research has yet to confirm this. Massage is also typically a part of these classes, which has been shown to strengthen the bond between caregiver and child as well as reduce stress in the child (Lee, 2006).

Tips for teaching yoga to infants or young toddlers
- Keep classes short, around 20–30 minutes.
- Keep class size small.
- Provide plenty of props such as blankets, blocks and cushions to make the class comfortable.
- Have mats and props set up before class.
- Make sure all postures allow the caregiver to keep physical contact with their child.
- Allow caregivers to feed or change a diaper during class.

EXAMPLE BABY YOGA SEQUENCE

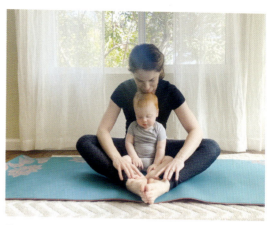

Figure 10.1 Double bound angle pose.

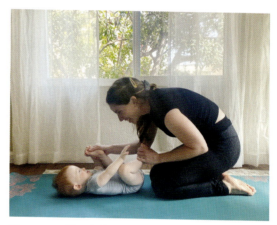

Figure 10.2 Bicycle legs with baby.

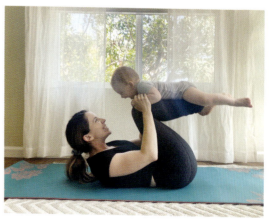

Figure 10.3 Leg lift with baby.

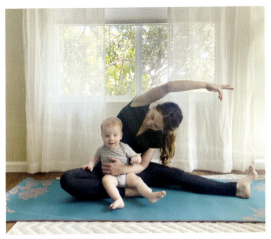
Figure 10.4 Seated side stretch variation.

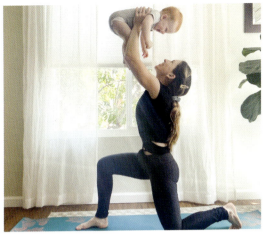
Figure 10.7 Low lunge with baby.

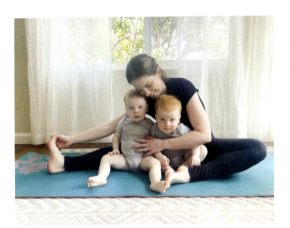
Figure 10.5 Leg stretch variation.

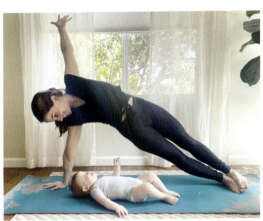
Figure 10.8 Side plank while looking at baby.

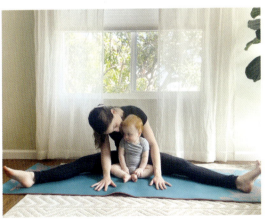
Figure 10.6 Seated forward fold.

Main takeaways
- The human brain goes through incredible growth during the first few years of life. The early years build the foundation for future brain health.
- Brain development is influenced by both genes and experiences.
- Yoga can help with muscle and nerve development. It may also improve sleep patterns and reduce levels of stress hormones, such as cortisol.

THE MATURING BRAIN: CHILDREN AND ADOLESCENTS

In childhood (ages 5–12) and adolescence (ages 12–18), the maturing brain starts to become more specialized to assume more complex functions. The brain continues to prune back unused or unneeded connections, but it also begins to become less capable of creating new connections between neurons (Cressman et al., 2010; Mallya et al., 2018). Although it is always possible to learn a new skill like a foreign language, it becomes more difficult as the brain matures.

Many brain changes occur during this time, including changes in brain structure and function. The social-emotional system that leads to increased reward-seeking becomes most active during puberty and declines during adulthood as the cognitive control system becomes more developed (Steinberg, 2008). The prefrontal cortex, which is part of the cognitive control system responsible for reasoning and behavioral control, is one of the last regions of the brain to reach maturity (Arain et al., 2013). Scientists believe this delay in prefrontal cortex maturity is what makes adolescents prone to impulsive behavior. The adolescent period is also when people start to form their identities and sense of self. This is an influential time, and the human brain is designed to remember memories most strongly from this period of life (Munawar, Kuhn and Haque, 2018).

The benefit of yoga and meditation for children and adolescents

Participating in regular exercise and meditation as a child impacts brain development. Yoga helps grow connections between neurons involved in balance and flexibility (Donahoe-Fillmore and Grant, 2019). Mindfulness meditation can improve academic performance and the ability to concentrate, reduce anxiety and depression, and improve social skills (Beauchemin, Hutchins and Patterson, 2008; Ching et al., 2015).

To harness the long-term benefits of yoga and meditation, it may make sense to start practicing at a young age. Researchers from Heidelberg University in Germany and the University of Sfax in Tunisia examined how a three-month yoga intervention impacted kindergarteners' cognitive performance, coordination and behavior (Jarraya et al., 2019). In the study, kindergarteners participated in Hatha yoga twice a week for 30 minutes, while another group of children participated in physical education, and a third group did no physical activity at all.

The kindergarteners who participated in the yoga condition showed increases in attention and coordination and less hyperactivity than the physical education group. The young yogis could also complete a task faster than the kids who participated in physical education or no exercise at all. The findings demonstrate that yoga may be a useful classroom tool that can help children learn to focus and self-regulate (Jarraya et al., 2019).

In 2016, researchers from Harvard Medical School and Kripalu Center for Yoga & Health conducted a review on how school-based yoga programs impact adolescents' mental, emotional, physical and behavioral health (Khalsa and Butzer, 2016). The scientists examined 47 publications on the topic and found that yoga improves all aspects of child and adolescent health in the school setting. They note that research in this field is limited and should be considered preliminary.

Mental health

The brain and other biological systems are most adaptable early in life. The development of resilience from an early age lays the foundation for a host of resilient behaviors for the rest of life. Contemplative practices can help kids become more resilient and cope with stress in positive ways. Yoga and meditation can improve mood, self-confidence, emotion regulation and resiliency (Hagen and Nayar, 2014). Thus, these practices are a helpful tool for improving health both physically and mentally.

Researchers from Rutgers University reviewed 27 studies looking at the effects of yoga as an intervention for children and adolescents with anxiety and depression (James-Palmer *et al.*, 2020). Although the type of yoga intervention varied across the different studies, 58 percent of the studies showed that yoga helped alleviate symptoms of both anxiety and depression. For studies that only examined the benefit of yoga on anxiety or depression, 70 percent of studies found improvement for symptoms of anxiety, while 40 percent showed decreased symptoms of depression. Despite the seemingly strong findings, the authors note that many of the studies were low to moderate quality (James-Palmer *et al.*, 2020). However, it does seem that yoga can lead to some level of reduction in symptomology for both anxiety and depression for children and adolescents.

Another systematic review explored different forms of exercise and how they affect students with attention deficit hyperactivity disorder (ADHD) (Cerrillo-Urbina *et al.*, 2015). The researchers, from the University of Castilla-La Mancha in Spain, included eight randomized control trials in their analysis with 249 total participants. When examining the results from the eight studies, the scientists found that yoga improved symptoms of ADHD, including inattention, hyperactivity and impulsivity (Cerrillo-Urbina *et al.*, 2015).

Another study conducted by scientists from Duke University found that a one-year interventional program that consisted of yoga, meditation and play therapy helped students aged 6–11 years old with ADHD improve their academic performance (Mehta *et al.*, 2012). The program also helped to decrease their symptoms of ADHD. Programs such as this one can be easily implemented in the school setting and should be considered a cost-effective option to aid students with ADHD.

Tips for teaching yoga to children and adolescents

- Create a yoga story for young children. Chose a theme and 5–8 yoga postures that can be incorporated into the story. Connect the postures, story and imagination to create a fun class!
- Young children generally have short attention spans of just a few minutes long. Thus, short meditations can help to engage their brain and boost their ability to concentrate.
- Adolescents can follow a similar style of class as an adult, but it's important to remember that their brains are still developing, and their attention spans are shorter.
- If you're teaching multiple adolescents in a class, you could consider incorporating some games or partner work. For example, you could use double tree pose to practice balancing with another person. These activities help develop interpersonal skills and cooperation.
- Incorporate music into the yoga routine for even more brain activation!

Example yoga story for young kids

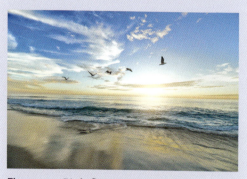

Figure 10.9 Birds flying over the beach.
Source: Frank McKenna on Unsplash.

Imagine you're walking down a sandy beach. Start to put sunscreen on your arms and try to reach around to get your back. Then you notice a seagull on your left. Can you show me what pose might look like a seagull? Good, now keep walking down the beach. You spot a seal playing in the waves. What pose might look like a seal? You keep walking down the beach and you start to feel a little sleepy from the strong sun. You lie down on your towel to rest.

the benefits lasted nearly seven weeks after the intervention.

Example mindfulness meditation for children

Find a comfortable seat or lie down.
Allow your eyes to close.
Start to listen to the sounds immediately around you.
What can you hear?
Now, start to listen to sounds that are a little further away.
Can you hear any birds or cars?
Try to listen to every sound around you.

Example breathing exercise for children and adolescents

Let's all sit down together.
Take a deep breath in.
Now, hold your breath for a count of four.
And blow the air out, making a "woosh" sound.
Let's try it again.
Repeat this exercise four times.

Mindfulness meditation is another contemplative practice that helps children learn about becoming more aware of their senses, improve their emotion regulation, develop compassion and connection, and promote social-emotional learning (Moreno-Gómez and Cejudo, 2018).

Mindfulness programs improve classroom behavior. In a large study of 409 elementary school students, scientists from the University of California, Los Angeles studied the effects of a five-week mindfulness program on various measures of behavior, including paying attention, self-control, participation in activities and respect for others (Black and Fernando, 2013). They found that student behavior was significantly improved from the intervention, and

Main takeaways

- In childhood and adolescence, the maturing brain starts to become more specialized to assume more complex functions.
- The prefrontal cortex is one of the last brain regions to reach maturity, which is why adolescents are prone to impulsive behavior.
- Yoga helps to grow connections between neurons involved in balance and flexibility.
- Yoga can also be a useful classroom tool that can help children and adolescents learn to focus and self-regulate.

- Practicing yoga may also help to reduce symptoms of anxiety and depression as well as improve symptoms of ADHD.

- Meditation can improve academic performance, the ability to concentrate, reduce anxiety and depression, and improve social skills.

BECOMING YOU: THE ADULT BRAIN

The twenties are transformative years of young adulthood. Although the brain reaches its adult volume by the age of ten, many regions of the brain have not yet reached full maturity. The brain matures from back to front. The occipital lobe is thought to mature around age 20, while the prefrontal cortex doesn't reach maturity until closer to 30 years old. As the brain's anatomy continues to change, so do its functions. Things like self-evaluation, long-term planning and emotion regulation become much easier. Decision making and judgment also begin to come into focus as the prefontal cortex comes fully online.

Yoga and meditation for adults

In general, yoga and meditation help improve and maintain physical and mental health by increasing quality of life and coping skills, decreasing stress, and improving self-compassion and blood pressure (Ditto, Eclache and Goldman, 2006; Nidich et al., 2009; Gard et al., 2012).

But inclusivity (or the lack of it) can be an issue in many studios. For example, yoga can positively impact body image, but it depends on the class environment. Participants in a study conducted by researchers from the University of Minnesota described yoga as having a positive impact on physical changes, gratitude for their body, self-confidence and a sense of accomplishment (Neumark-Sztainer, Watts and Rydell, 2018). The yogis also described how classes sometimes felt competitive as they looked around the room and saw a lack of diversity in body shapes and sizes practicing yoga. Men also do not often see themselves represented in the studio setting. Yoga studios and instructors should try to provide an inclusive environment for yogis of all shapes, sizes, genders, orientations and abilities.

Tips for making a yoga class more inclusive
- Normalize and provide variations for postures that will work for a wide range of bodies and abilities.
- Use language that is without judgment and not competitive.
- Cue using words like "invite" or "explore" to encourage students to try a pose or movements.
- Ask students to inquire about their own feelings during practice instead of telling them how to feel.
- Keep language gender-neutral to allow for a wide range of experiences. Try "welcome everyone" instead of "welcome ladies" when greeting the class, and find ways to cue body landmarks without referring to gendered parts.

Adapted from: Making Yoga More Inclusive: Language Do's and Don'ts by Amber Karnes. From: https://yogainternational.com/article/view/inclusive-yoga

The modern world has also brought forth a host of new challenges. Due to the demands of technology and multitasking, people often struggle with sustained attention and working memory. Scientists at the University of California, San Francisco wanted to create a meditation program to help young adults improve their attention and memory (Ziegler *et al.*, 2019). They created a tablet-based, six-week focused-attention meditation program called MediTrain. Consistent use of the program led to gains in both sustained attention and working memory in the participants. The researchers also observed changes in the participants' brain waves related to attentional control, suggesting that a technology-based meditation program may be a feasible means of enhancing attention.

Main takeaways
- The brain matures from back to front. The occipital lobe is thought to mature around age 20, while the prefrontal cortex doesn't reach maturity until closer to 30 years old.
- Yoga can be beneficial for both physical and mental health; however, it is important to make sure the class is inclusive.
- Tablet-based meditation programs may be helpful for increasing attention and working memory, which can both be compromised due to multitasking.

HEALTHY AGING: THE AGING BRAIN

Staying cognitively engaged and exercising throughout the lifespan activates neurons and nerves, keeping them healthy by improving blood flow and stimulation. As the brain gets older, it starts to shrink as brain cells die. Physical exercise (such as yoga), brain exercises (like meditation) and a healthy diet may offer significant protection against this decline.

Regular exercise can protect the brain from decline. According to the Centers for Disease Control and Prevention, it is recommended that the average adult participate in aerobic exercise for at least 30 minutes five days a week and work on strength training at least two days a week (CDC, 2022). Aerobic activity is anything that causes the breath to increase and makes the heart beat faster. Strength training is physical activity that focuses on strengthening the muscles. Some yoga classes like Power Yoga and Vinyasa yoga incorporate both aerobic exercises and strength training using the weight of the body to provide a multitude of brain-boosting benefits.

Why is exercise so good for us? Exercise increases the heart rate, which improves blood flow throughout the body, including the brain. Increased blood flow means more nutrients are circulating to the brain. Movement helps reduce inflammation, which is implicated in many neurological conditions, such as multiple sclerosis and Alzheimer's disease. Exercise also tends to reduce emotional stress, which decreases the levels of stress hormones circulating in your body.

Exercise can:

- reduce symptoms of anxiety and depression
- improve sleep and cognition
- help with weight management
- lead to stronger bones and muscles
- reduce the risk of numerous conditions such as heart disease, stroke, diabetes and cancer
- increase lifespan and add years of healthy living (healthspan).

Exercise and the brain

Exercise impacts the brain on a molecular and cellular level. For example, exercise promotes processes that support brain remodeling called neuroplasticity (Huang *et al.*, 2021). Exercise can reduce the risk of developing cognitive decline and dementia, as well as slow down neurodegeneration in conditions like Alzheimer's disease (Lin, Tsai and Kuo, 2018).

Exercise also helps increase brain volume (gray matter) in areas like the hippocampus (Erickson, Leckie and Weinstein, 2014). Although the research is still preliminary, it appears that exercise may influence brain volume well into late adulthood (Erickson, Leckie and Weinstein, 2014). Yoga and meditation are also considered to be neuroprotective and can stall symptoms of aging.

Neurogenesis: creating new neurons in the brain

The brain may be able to produce new neurons late into life in a process called **neurogenesis**. For decades, neuroscientists did not believe that the adult brain could produce new neurons. The established dogma was that the human brain couldn't generate new neurons after birth (Gage, 2019).

In 1998, neuroscientist Rusty Gage made the discovery that the human brain can create new neurons in certain brain regions throughout the lifespan (Eriksson *et al.*, 1998). Specifically, his team found that neural stem cells, which become neurons, exist in the adult hippocampus.

Gage's work further showed that physical exercise can increase the brain's ability to generate more neurons (van Praag, 2005). His team examined the brains of mice who voluntarily ran on a wheel versus those who did not have access to a wheel. The older mice who ran on their wheels showed better cognition and problem solving than the sedentary mice. The active mice also showed more neurogenesis than the inactive mice. The study is one of the first to demonstrate that exercise (running, in this case) can help to slow the effects of aging on the brain.

However, not everyone agrees with Gage's findings. Arturo Alvarez-Buylla, a neuroscientist who also studies neurogenesis, argues that neurogenesis does not exist in adult humans (Sorrells *et al.*, 2018). Alvarez-Buylla has extensively examined neuron production in the hippocampus in both children and adults and found that neurogenesis declines sharply during the first year of life. His research has shown that by the time a person is 18 years old there is no trace of neurogenesis at all. Additionally, Alvarez-Buylla duplicated these findings in macaques, which further supports his claims.

An independent group of researchers at Yale University published a study demonstrating that mouse, pig and monkey (specifically macaques) brains showed some evidence of neurogenesis in the hippocampus while humans did not (Franjic *et al.*, 2022).

So, why can't neuroscientists agree? The human brain is incredibly difficult to study while the person is still alive. Many studies of neurogenesis rely on postmortem brains from people who have dedicated their bodies to science, but when the blood stops flowing, the brain shuts down. Thus, processes that had been occurring while the person was alive may no longer occur by the time the scientist acquires the brain.

Current methodologies available to study the brain are another limitation. It is possible that some of the chemicals used to identify neurogenesis may not be targeting the right proteins. New methods will likely need to be developed to truly understand and evaluate neurogenesis in the adult human brain.

Yoga may protect the brain

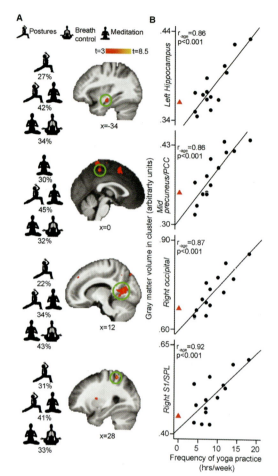

Figure 10.10 Certain brain regions were associated with the frequency of yoga-associated practices. For example, gray matter volume was related to the frequency of yoga practice in the left hippocampus. Thus, those who practiced the most often showed the largest hippocampal volumes, suggesting that yoga may offer some level of neuroprotection against aging.

Source: Villemure et al., 2015, originally published by Frontiers, CC BY 4.0. From: https://www.frontiersin.org/articles/10.3389/fnhum.2015.00281/full

Yoga may protect the brain from the cell death that is associated with aging. Scientists from the National Institutes of Health and McGill University in Canada examined the age-related benefits of yoga in experienced practitioners compared with a healthy control group (Villemure et al., 2015). In the study, they used structural magnetic resonance imaging (MRI) to take a closer look at gray matter differences between the groups.

In the control group, which consisted of 14 physically active participants, the scientists found that gray matter was lower in the older participants than in the younger participants, which was the expected result. Surprisingly, the yoga group, which also had 14 participants, showed no relationship between gray matter and age. Instead, gray matter in certain brain regions was related to the number of years of yoga practice as well as the weekly amount of yoga practice (Figure 10.10). Thus, the longer and more regularly the person practiced yoga, the larger the brain regions appeared (Villemure et al., 2015). These results suggest that yoga may offer a neuroprotective effect on the brain.

Yoga and meditation for memory and cognition

Aging is a physiological process that is marked by cognitive decline, usually affecting the brain's memory and executive function center, but contemplative practices are thought to slow or prevent this decline. The United States National Health Interview Survey asked adults why they practiced yoga, and over 30 percent responded that they practiced yoga to improve memory or concentration. Yoga and meditation are linked with improvements in both cognition and memory in older adults (Pandya, 2018; Prakash et al., 2012; Brandmeyer, Delorme and Wahbeh, 2019).

Scientists from Wayne State University and the University of Illinois examined the effect of a two-month Hatha yoga intervention on executive function, attention and processing speed in 118 older adults (Gothe, Kramer and McAuley, 2014, 2017). The scientists also included a stretching control group for comparison. They found that the yoga group showed significantly faster reaction times, working memory and executive function than the control group after the intervention. The yoga group also had improved cognitive processing and pattern comparison, suggesting that practicing Hatha yoga regularly could lead to cognitive benefits during the aging process. And these benefits are greater than just stretching alone (Gothe, Kramer and McAuley, 2014, 2017).

The Sanskrit effect
Many types of contemplative practices involve memorizing and repeating a specific mantra, such as oral texts in Sanskrit. Neuroscientists from the University of Trento in Italy wondered if this practice could enhance thinking and memory (Hartzell et al., 2016).

To study the "Sanskrit effect" on the brain, the scientists recruited Vedic pandits (Hindu scholars who train to memorize oral texts) from schools around Delhi, India and matched them with controls with the same age, gender, handedness, eye-dominance and multilingualism. Then, they used brain imaging to look for differences in the size of various brain regions between the two groups.

The scientists found that the pandits had multiple brain regions, including the hippocampus, that were much larger than those of the matched controls. Overall, the pandits also had about 10 percent more gray matter, which contains the neuronal cell bodies, than the controls across both hemispheres of the brain. The researchers believe more gray matter could be related to enhanced cognitive function (Hartzell et al., 2016). Next, the researchers plan to examine if the pandits' increase in hippocampus volume could help to stall the effects of Alzheimer's disease.

Another study conducted by researchers at the University of California, Los Angeles explored the effect of yoga on cognitive decline, while looking at connectivity between neurons (Eyre et al., 2016). Participants in the study were at least 55 years old and had mild cognitive impairment. Mild cognitive impairment is more serious cognitive decline than typically occurs during aging, but less severe than that observed in dementia. It is characterized by issues with memory, language or cognition. In the study, 14 participants were assigned to the yoga intervention and 11 participants were assigned to the memory enhancement training. Both interventions lasted for three months. Brain imaging was then used to map the relationship between brain networks and memory performance.

The scientists found that the yoga group demonstrated significant improvements in visual and spatial memory and levels of depression when compared with the memory task control group. Improved verbal memory performance was associated with an increase in connectivity between multiple brain networks, the cingulate cortex, the frontal cortex and the occipital cortex. Improved verbal memory performance was correlated with an increase in connectivity between the language processing network and a small part of the frontal cortex called the inferior frontal gyrus. The underlying mechanisms for the cognitive improvement are unknown, but it could be due to the increase in blood flow (and thus nutrients and oxygen) that occurs during movement practices.

Brain networks
Meditation may offer another possibility for facilitating healthy aging. One of the brain networks affected by aging is the default mode network, which is associated with mind wandering, self-reflection and interoception (the ability to sense the body's internal state). The default mode network is activated when a person is not engaged in a task or activity and becomes less active when the brain is engaged in a goal-directed task, like meditation.

Roughly 80–90 percent of the brain's energy

is used when the default mode network is active and the brain is not conducting any specific tasks (Chen and Zhang, 2021). Thus, the brain is processing high volumes of information, requiring lots of energy, even when it is not formally engaged in a task. The default mode network involves simultaneous activation of various brain regions, including part of the prefrontal cortex, the posterior cingulate cortex, the precuneus, and parts of the parietal and temporal lobes (Ramírez-Barrantes et al., 2019). When the default mode network becomes less active, another network called the **dorsal attention network** becomes more active. The dorsal attention network is involved in focused attention (Devaney et al., 2021).

Researchers from Harvard Medical School and Boston University used brain imaging to examine the differences in network activations between experienced Vipassana meditators (focused attention meditation) and matched controls (Devaney et al., 2021). The participants performed two attention tasks during the scan, while the scientists looked at which regions of the brain were being used. By examining which brain region became activated, the researchers found that the experienced meditators were able to regulate their default mode and dorsal attention networks significantly better than the control group (Devaney et al., 2021).

The scientists also scanned the participants' brains during rest to look at the connectivity between different brain regions. Once again, the meditators could more easily switch between their default mode and dorsal attention networks than the control group (Devaney et al., 2021). Similar to how the sympathetic and the parasympathetic nervous systems work together to provide the body with balance, the default mode and the dorsal attention networks help maintain homeostasis and brain health. The flexibility of being able to switch between the default mode and the dorsal attention networks is likely a long-term health benefit of meditation practice (Devaney et al., 2021).

Being able to regulate the default mode network could also provide a neuroprotective effect against aging (Ramírez-Barrantes et al., 2019). Meditation increases meta-awareness, a cognitive ability that involves the default mode network. Although there are many types of meditation, most of them involve a steady, relaxed focus on the present moment.

A study conducted by researchers at the University of Massachusetts and Yale University also found that meditation leads to reduced default mode network activity long after the meditation task (Garrison et al., 2015). This finding suggests that the brain stays in a focused state after the meditation is finished and may explain why meditation helps curb mind wandering and self-related thinking (Garrison et al., 2015).

Decreased default mode network activity is related to improved cognitive performance, whereas increased default mode network activity is associated with a multitude of mental health conditions, including anxiety, depression and addiction (Coutinho et al., 2015; Zhang and Volkow, 2019). Mind wandering is a major feature of many of these conditions, especially anxiety (Seli et al., 2019). Thus, meditation could help promote mental health and improve cognitive function.

Considerations for older yogis

The proprioception and vestibular systems change during aging, which can cause dizziness and issues with balance (Piitulainen et al., 2018). These changes put older adults at an increased risk for falls and injuries. Roughly 30 percent of individuals over the age of 60 experience these symptoms (Brosel and Strupp, 2019).

Safety is the priority when designing yoga classes for older adults. Consider classes that offer a slower pace with more emphasis on form, such as gentle, restorative, or chair yoga. Chair yoga is becoming popular in the United States for older adults, those with health conditions and those recovering from injuries. Many studios and online streaming services offer chair yoga classes.

EXAMPLE CHAIR YOGA SEQUENCE FOR OLDER ADULTS

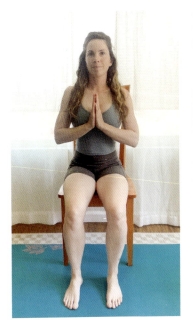

Figure 10.11 Seated prayer pose.

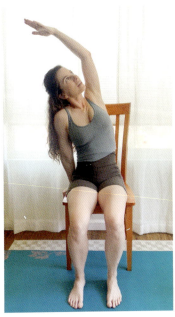

Figure 10.13 Seated side stretch.

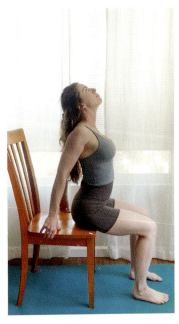

Figure 10.15 Cow pose variation with arm support.

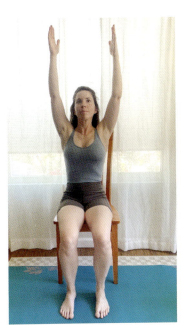

Figure 10.12 Arm extension above the head.

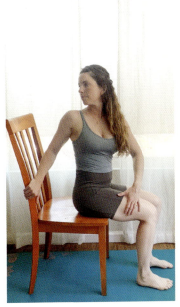

Figure 10.14 Supported spinal twist.

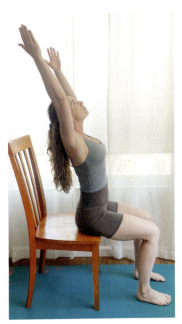

Figure 10.16 Chest opener variation.

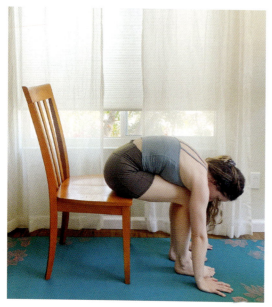

Figure 10.17 Seated forward fold.

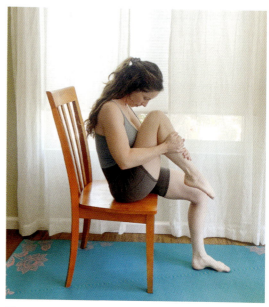

Figure 10.19 Nose to knee pose.

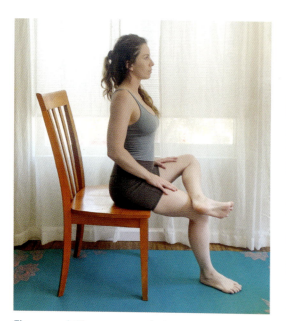

Figure 10.18 Pigeon pose variation.

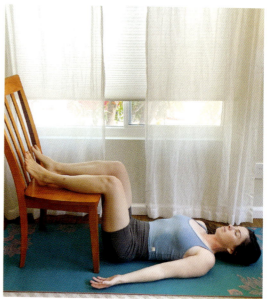

Figure 10.20 Corpse pose variation using a chair to lift and support the legs.

Researchers are currently examining how individual postures impact older adults. In a recent study, scientists at the University of Southern California used biomechanical methods to examine the joint angles, force and muscle activity of 21 Hatha yoga postures in 20 adults with an average age of 70 (Salem *et al.*, 2013). The scientists found that certain postures put repetitive loading on the same joints and muscles. While some postures were more difficult, the modifications were not always intuitive. Their findings highlight the importance of providing a balanced yoga routine with a variety of postures as well as offering explicit and accessible modifications during class. Studies like this one may help to guide more effective yoga programs in the future.

> **Main takeaways**
> - Yoga, meditation and a healthy diet may offer significant protection against cognitive decline related to aging.
> - Exercise increases the heart rate which improves blood flow throughout the body, including the brain. Better blood flow increases the circulation of nutrients and reduces inflammation.
> - The brain may be able to produce new neurons late into life in a process called **neurogenesis**. However, neurogenesis likely only occurs in the hippocampus, if at all.
> - Yoga and meditation are linked with improvements in both cognition and memory in older adults.
> - Practicing meditation can help individuals to regulate their attentional and resting state brain networks, which may be neuroprotective against aging.
> - Safety is the priority when designing yoga classes for older adults as their proprioception and vestibular systems change during aging, which can cause dizziness and issues with balance.

THE YOGIC DIET AND BRAIN HEALTH

Contemplative practices are associated with a healthier lifestyle. Those who practice yoga and meditation are often health-focused, which may have led them to practice yoga and meditation in the first place. Additionally, the yogic concept of "do no harm" leads many to eat fewer animal products, so as to not harm animals and the environment. Eating a diet full of whole, unprocessed foods has a host of health benefits, including lowering cholesterol, body weight, blood pressure and blood sugar; reducing the risk of cancer and diabetes; reversing atherosclerosis; decreasing inflammation in the body; and improving psychological wellness by making healthier choices (Barnard *et al.*, 2019).

Food for your brain: the MIND diet

A lot of research has been conducted on the best diet for brain health, and one of the most popular and successful nutrition plans is the MIND diet. The MIND diet, created by researchers at Harvard University and Rush University, is a plant-based diet that focuses on minimally or non-processed foods. The diet revolves around eating whole grains (like quinoa or oats), fruits, vegetables, legumes, nuts and berries. Poultry and fish can be eaten once a week, and olive oil should be used instead of butter.

Researchers have shown that by following the MIND diet, there is a reduced risk of developing dementia, Alzheimer's disease and other age-related forms of cognitive decline (Morris et al., 2015a,b; Berendsen et al., 2017). Foods like kale, spinach and collard greens are packed with nutrients, such as folate, vitamin E and flavonoids, that are thought to slow brain aging. Eating berries, such as blueberries and strawberries, has also been shown to reduce the rate of cognitive decline (Devore et al., 2012). Nuts are another nutrient-rich food packed with vitamin E that exhibit brain-protective qualities. Foods that are high in protein and fiber, such as beans, lentils and soybeans, are high in B vitamins that help keep the brain healthy.

> **Tips for getting started**
> - Start with "Meatless Mondays" and try to cook a plant-based meal every Monday.
> - Purchase a healthy eating cookbook for inspiration.
> - Find an accountability partner that you can check in with about your healthy eating progress.
> - Use frozen fruits and vegetables for cooking when you're in a rush. They're often flash frozen, which helps preserve their nutrients.
> - Make an action plan about your eating that includes what and when you're going to make plant-based meals.

Eating for health and ahimsa

Many elite athletes, such as tennis stars Serena and Venus Williams, ultramarathon runner Scott Jurek and bodybuilder Patrik Baboumian, have switched to plant-based diets to increase their athletic performance. Following a plant-based diet can decrease weight and body fat percentage as well as enhance athletic endurance (Barnard et al., 2005, 2019). Yoga practitioners who are taking or teaching multiple classes a day or those who participate in longer classes may benefit from plant-based eating. Plant-based diets help improve cardiovascular health, which is critical for pumping blood, nutrients and oxygen throughout the body (Kim et al., 2019).

Plant-based diets also help with recovery by reducing systemic inflammation (Barnard et al., 2019; Naclerio et al., 2020). Exercise produces byproducts called free radicals that cause inflammation, especially with vigorous exercise. A buildup of free radicals, called oxidative stress, can lead to cell and tissue damage over time. A balanced plant-based diet is filled with antioxidants that can help to reduce this inflammation and lead to faster recovery.

Eating fewer animal products and practicing yoga also have philosophical overlap. For example, in *The Yoga Sutras of Patanjali*, Patanjali lists the eight limbs of yoga, which are the ethical guidelines of living. The eight limbs include the yamas (things to avoid) and the niyamas (things to do). Following the eight limbs is thought to bring the yogi closer to enlightenment and connection with the world.

One of the yamas is called ahimsa or nonviolence. The concept of ahimsa translates to doing no harm to others, both physically and verbally, and many believe this includes animals. One way to practice nonviolence towards animals is to consume fewer or no animal products.

> **Main takeaways**
> - Eating a diet full of whole, unprocessed foods has a host of health benefits, including lowering cholesterol, body weight, blood pressure and blood sugar.
> - The MIND diet can help to reduce the risk of developing dementia, Alzheimer's disease and other age-related forms of cognitive decline.
> - Plant-based diets can help with recovery by reducing systemic inflammation.

THE NEUROSCIENCE OF SLEEP AND YOGA NIDRA

With age, sleep patterns begin to change. Sleep not only affects the brain, but it affects how the body ages. Studies have shown that sleeping for short periods at night is associated with age-related brain cell death and cognitive decline in older adults (Gorgoni and De Gennaro, 2021). Sleep deprivation can cause changes in brain plasticity and cognitive function.

Circadian rhythms also become less coordinated with age, and daytime napping becomes more common (Gorgoni and De Gennaro, 2021). Aging can spur impaired quality and quantity of sleep, but yogic sleep called yoga nidra, discussed below, may offer benefits to those with sleep problems.

What is sleep?
The average person spends approximately one third of their life sleeping, which is equivalent to 33 years sleeping if they live to 100 years old (Kraftl and Horton, 2008). Scientists only partially understand why humans need sleep, and they are currently exploring what is occurring during sleep on a molecular level. Despite this gap in scientific knowledge, sleep is clearly necessary for functioning as sleep deprivation can lead to death.

Circadian rhythms regulate the sleep–wake cycle and occur every 24 hours. This process involves a few regions of the brain, including the hypothalamus and the pineal gland. When light hits the eye, signals are sent to a group of neurons in the hypothalamus called the suprachiasmatic nucleus (Figure 10.21). If the eyes perceive darkness, then the suprachiasmatic neurons tell the pineal gland to produce melatonin to promote falling asleep. During sleep, neurons send signals to each other in wave patterns. The different wave patterns of signals represent the four different stages of sleep (Figure 10.22) and can be measured by researchers using an electroencephalogram or EEG.

The first two stages involve light sleep. The third stage of sleep is deep sleep, and it is thought to be important for rest and recovery. The final stage is called rapid eye movement (REM) sleep. During REM sleep, the eyes move quickly, as the muscles relax and dreaming occurs. It is also very difficult to wake during REM sleep.

The brain moves through all four stages of sleep multiple times throughout the night. Although scientists have not figured out exactly *why* sleep is important for health, recent research suggests that sleep may be the time when the brain repairs damage and flushes out toxins (Cao *et al.*, 2020). Sleep may also be a period when the brain strengthens pathways to solidify memories (Stickgold, 2005).

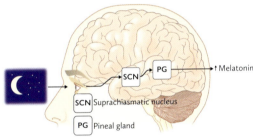

Figure 10.21 When the eyes perceive darkness, neurons in the suprachiasmatic nucleus of the hypothalamus send signals to the pineal gland. The pineal gland then produces melatonin to promote falling asleep.

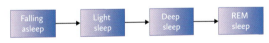

Figure 10.22 The four main stages of sleep, which include falling asleep, light sleep, deep sleep and REM sleep.

Meditation for sleep
Meditation is a beneficial tool for improving sleep (Ong *et al.*, 2014). One form of meditation called **yoga nidra** has been shown to be especially effective in promoting sleep and relaxation while decreasing stress and anxiety (Sharpe *et al.*, 2020; Moszeik, von Oertzen and Renner, 2020; Dol, 2019). Yoga nidra, also known as yogic sleep,

is typically performed lying down in savasana (corpse pose) while a teacher guides the student through states of relaxation and sleep using the voice (Parker, Bharati and Fernandez, 2013).

It does not take a lot of meditation practice to see results. Studies have shown that even one hour of yoga nidra twice a week can significantly decrease symptoms of stress and improve self-esteem (Dol, 2019). Yoga nidra may also be slightly more effective at reducing symptoms of anxiety than seated forms of meditation (Ferreira-Vorkapic et al., 2018).

Numerous yoga nidra studies have been conducted using a form of yogic sleep called iRest. Developed by researcher and clinical psychologist Richard Miller, iRest is a "meditation practice based on the ancient tradition of yoga nidra and adapted to suit the conditions of modern life" (iRest, 2022). iRest can alleviate symptoms of depression and anxiety in addition to improving sleep (Wahbeh and Nelson, 2019; Livingston and Collette-Merrill, 2018). It is also currently approved by the United States military to be used as a complementary and alternative medicine for post-traumatic stress disorder and pain management (Livingston and Collette-Merrill, 2018).

Yoga nidra

Lie down in a comfortable position. Allow the eyes to close and gently close your mouth, if accessible, and start to breathe in and out through the nose. Bring your focus to the sounds of the world around you. Visualize your body resting on the ground and become aware of your physical presence.

Now, start to move inward, inside your body. Find the inner place where you feel calm and secure. Spend a moment bathing in the feelings of this inner haven. You can return to this place at any point in this practice. It is here. It is yours. Slowly, start to bring your awareness back to your physical body. Feel your entire, connected physical presence on the floor. Feel the breath enter your body through the nostrils. Try to follow the breath as it moves down your trachea into your lungs and then back up and out the nostrils. Feel energized by the inhale and invite relaxation with the exhale. Without any judgment, bring awareness to any emotions or feelings that you are experiencing in the current moment. Acknowledge any tension or stress. And then try to bring forth that feeling of inner calm you experienced before. Allow the peace to replace the stress. Let the stress flow out of the body. Now bring forth a memory that holds joy. Notice the details of this memory and allow it to fill you with warmth.

Linger in this warmth. Soak it up. Once again, start to come back to the breath. Back into the physical body. Notice how your body feels. Become aware of the room around you and how your body fits into the space. When you are ready, start to wiggle your fingers and toes, coming back into the present moment. Welcome back.

Main takeaways

- Sleep changes as we get older and can affect how we feel and age.
- The brain moves through four stages of sleep multiple times throughout the night.
- Scientists believe that sleep may be the time when the brain repairs damage and flushes out toxins.
- **Yoga nidra** can promote sleep and relaxation while decreasing stress and anxiety.

REFERENCES

Arain, M., Haque, M., Johal, L., Mathur, P., et al., 2013. Maturation of the adolescent brain. *Neuropsychiatric Disease and Treatment*, 9, pp.449–461.

Barnard, N. Goldman, D.M., Loomis, J.F., Kahleova, H., et al., 2019. Plant-based diets for cardiovascular safety and performance in endurance sports. *Nutrients*, 11(1), p.130.

Barnard, N.D., Scialli, A.R., Turner-McGrievy, G., Lanou, A.J., & Glass, J., 2005. The effects of a low-fat, plant-based dietary intervention on body weight, metabolism, and insulin sensitivity. *The American Journal of Medicine*, 118(9), pp.991–997.

Beauchemin, J., Hutchins, T.L., & Patterson, F., 2008. Mindfulness meditation may lessen anxiety, promote social skills, and improve academic performance among adolescents with learning disabilities. *Complementary Health Practice Review*, 13(1), pp.34–45.

Berendsen, A.M., Kang, J.H., Feskens, E.J.M., de Groot, C.P.G.M., Grodstein, F., & van de Rest, O., 2017. Association of long-term adherence to the MIND diet with cognitive function and cognitive decline in American women. *The Journal of Nutrition, Health & Aging*, 22(2), pp.222–229.

Black, D.S., & Fernando, R., 2013. Mindfulness training and classroom behavior among lower-income and ethnic minority elementary school children. *Journal of Child and Family Studies*, 23(7), pp.1242–1246.

Brandmeyer, T., Delorme, A., & Wahbeh, H., 2019. The neuroscience of meditation: classification, phenomenology, correlates, and mechanisms. *Progress in Brain Research*, 244, pp.1–29.

Brosel, S., & Strupp, M., 2019. The vestibular system and ageing. *Subcellular Biochemistry*, 91, pp.195–225.

Cao, J., Herman, A.B., West, G.B., Pao, G., & Savage, V.M., 2020. Unraveling why we sleep: quantitative analysis reveals abrupt transition from neural reorganization to repair in early development. *Science Advances*, 6(38), eaba0398.

Centers for Disease Control and Prevention (CDC), 2022. How much physical activity do adults need? Available at: www.cdc.gov/physicalactivity/basics/adults/index.htm

Cerrillo-Urbina, A.J., García-Hermoso, A., Sánchez-López, M., Pardo-Guijarro, M.J., Santos Gómez, J.L., & Martínez-Vizcaíno, V., 2015. The effects of physical exercise in children with attention deficit hyperactivity disorder: a systematic review and meta-analysis of randomized control trials. *Child: Care, Health and Development*, 41(6), pp.779–788.

Chen, Y., & Zhang, J., 2021. How energy supports our brain to yield consciousness: insights from neuroimaging based on the neuroenergetics hypothesis. *Frontiers in Systems Neuroscience*, 15, 648860.

Ching, H.-H., Koo, M., Tsai, T.-H., & Chen, C.-Y., 2015. Effects of a mindfulness meditation course on learning and cognitive performance among university students in Taiwan. *Evidence-Based Complementary and Alternative Medicine*, 2015, pp.1–7.

Coutinho, J.F., Fernandes, S.V., Soares, J.M., Maia, L., Gonçalves, Ó.F., & Sampaio, A., 2015. Default mode network dissociation in depressive and anxiety states. *Brain Imaging and Behavior*, 10(1), pp.147–157.

Cressman, V.L., Balaban, J., Steinfeld, S., Shemyakin, A., et al., 2010. Prefrontal cortical inputs to the basal amygdala undergo pruning during late adolescence in the rat. *The Journal of Comparative Neurology*, 518(14), pp.2693–2709.

Devaney, K., Levin, E.J., Tripathi, V., Higgins, J.P., Lazar, S.W., & Somers, D.C., 2021. Attention and default mode network assessments of meditation experience during active cognition and rest. *Brain Sciences*, 11(5), p.566.

Devore, E.E., Kang, J.H., Breteler, M.M.B., & Grodstein, F., et al., 2012. Dietary intakes of berries and flavonoids in relation to cognitive decline. *Annals of Neurology*, 72(1), pp.135–143.

Ditto, B., Eclache, M., & Goldman, N., 2006. Short-term autonomic and cardiovascular effects of mindfulness body scan meditation. *Annals of Behavioral Medicine*, 32(3), pp.227–234.

Dol, K.S., 2019. Effects of a yoga nidra on the life stress and self-esteem in university students. *Complementary Therapies in Clinical Practice*, 35, pp.232–236.

Donahoe-Fillmore, B., & Grant, E., 2019. The effects of yoga practice on balance, strength, coordination and flexibility in healthy children aged 10–12 years. *Journal of Bodywork and Movement Therapies*, 23(4), pp.708–712.

Erickson, K.I., Leckie, R.L., & Weinstein, A.M., 2014. Physical activity, fitness, and gray matter volume. *Neurobiology of Aging*, 35(Supplement 2), S20–S28.

Eriksson, P.S., Perfilieva, E., Björk-Eriksson, T., Albron, A.-M., et al., 1998. Neurogenesis in the adult human hippocampus. *Nature Medicine*, 4(11), pp.1313–1317.

Eyre, H.A., Acevedo, B., Yang, H., Siddarth, P., et al., 2016. Changes in neural connectivity and memory following a yoga intervention for older adults: a pilot study. *Journal of Alzheimer's Disease*, 52(2), pp.673–684.

Ferreira-Vorkapic, C., Borba-Pinheiro, C.J., Marchioro, M., & Santana, D., 2018. The impact of yoga nidra and seated meditation on the mental health of college professors. *International Journal of Yoga*, 11(3), p.215.

Franjic, D., Skarica, M., Ma, S., Arellano, J.I., et al., 2022. Transcriptomic taxonomy and neurogenic trajectories of adult human, macaque, and pig hippocampal and entorhinal cells. *Neuron*, 110(3), pp.452–469.e14.

Gage, F.H., 2019. Adult neurogenesis in mammals. *Science*, 364(6443), pp.827–828.

Gard, T., Brach N., Hölzel, B.K., Noggle, J.J., Conboy, L.A., & Lazar, S.W., 2012. Effects of a yoga-based intervention for young adults on quality of life and perceived stress: the potential mediating roles of mindfulness and self-compassion. *The Journal of Positive Psychology*, 7(3), pp.165–175.

Garrison, K.A., Zeffiro, T.A., Scheinost, D., Constable, R.T., & Brewer, J.A., 2015. Meditation leads to reduced default mode network activity beyond an active task. *Cognitive, Affective, & Behavioral Neuroscience*, 15(3), pp.712–720.

Gilmore, J.H., Knickmeyer, R.C., & Gao, W., 2018. Imaging structural and functional brain development in early childhood. *Nature Reviews Neuroscience*, 19(3), pp.123–137.

Gorgoni, M., & De Gennaro, L., 2021. Sleep in the aging brain. *Brain Sciences*, 11(2), p.229.

Gothe, N.P., Kramer, A.F., & McAuley, E., 2014. The effects of an 8-week Hatha yoga intervention on executive function in older adults. *The Journals of Gerontology: Series A*, 69(9), pp.1109–1116.

Gothe, N.P., Kramer, A.F., & McAuley, E., 2017. Hatha yoga practice improves attention and processing speed in older adults: results from an 8-week randomized control trial. *The Journal of Alternative and Complementary Medicine*, 23(1), pp.35–40.

Hagen, I., & Nayar, U.S., 2014. Yoga for children and young people's mental health and well-being: research review and reflections on the mental health potentials of yoga. *Frontiers in Psychiatry*, 5, p.35.

Hartzell, J.F., Davis, B., Melcher, D., Miceli, G. et al., 2016. Brains of verbal memory specialists show anatomical differences in language, memory and visual systems. *NeuroImage*, 131, pp.181–192.

Harvard University, 2007. The science of early childhood development. Center on the Developing Child at Harvard University. Available at: https://developingchild.harvard.edu/resources/inbrief-science-of-ecd/

Huang, Z., Zhang, Y., Zhou, R., Yang, L., & Pan, H., et al., 2021. Lactate as potential mediators for exercise-induced positive effects on neuroplasticity and cerebrovascular plasticity. *Frontiers in Physiology*, 12, 656455.

Ikeda, K., & Teasdale, H., 2018. Why you can't remember being a baby. Queensland Brain Institute. Available at: https://qbi.uq.edu.au/brain/learning-memory/why-you-cant-remember-being-baby

iRest, 2022. About iRest. Available at: www.irest.org/about-irest

James-Palmer, A., Anderson, E.Z., Zucker, L., Kofman, Y., & Daneault, J.-F., et al., 2020. Yoga as an intervention for the reduction of symptoms of anxiety and depression in children and adolescents: a systematic review. *Frontiers in Pediatrics*, 8, p.78.

Jarraya, S., Wagner, M., Jarraya, M., & Engel, F.A., 2019. 12 weeks of kindergarten-based yoga practice increases visual attention, visual-motor precision and decreases behavior of inattention and hyperactivity in 5-year-old children. *Frontiers in Psychology*, 10, p.796.

Khalsa, S.B., & Butzer, B., 2016. Yoga in school settings: a research review. *Annals of the New York Academy of Sciences*, 1373(1), pp.45–55.

Kim, H., Caulfield, L.E., Garcia-Larsen, V., Steffen, L.M., Coresh, J., & Rebholz, C.M., 2019. Plant-based diets are associated with a lower risk of incident cardiovascular disease, cardiovascular disease mortality, and all-cause mortality in a general population of middle-aged adults. *Journal of the American Heart Association*, 8(16), e012865.

Kraftl, P., & Horton, J., 2008. Spaces of every-night life: for geographies of sleep, sleeping and sleepiness. *Progress in Human Geography*, 32(4), pp.509–524.

Lee, H.K., 2006. The effects of infant massage on weight, height, and mother–infant interaction. *Journal of Korean Academy of Nursing*, 36(8), p.1331.

Lin, T.-W., Tsai, S.-F., & Kuo, Y.-M., 2018. Physical exercise enhances neuroplasticity and delays Alzheimer's disease. *Brain Plasticity*, 4(1), pp.95–110.

Livingston, E., & Collette-Merrill, K., 2018. Effectiveness of Integrative Restoration (iRest) yoga nidra on mindfulness, sleep, and pain in health care workers. *Holistic Nursing Practice*, 32(3), pp.160–166.

MacDonald, C., 2013. Mother and baby yoga is good for you. *The Practicing Midwife*, 16(5), pp.14, 16, 18.

Mallya, A.P., Wang, H.-D., Lee, H.N.R., & Deutch, A.Y., 2018. Microglial pruning of synapses in the prefrontal cortex during adolescence. *Cerebral Cortex*, 29(4), pp.1634–1643.

Mehta, S., Shah, D., Shah, K., Mehta, S. et al., 2012. Peer-mediated multimodal intervention program for the treatment of children with ADHD in India: one-year followup. *ISRN Pediatrics*, 2012, pp.1–7.

Moreno-Gómez, A.-J., & Cejudo, J., 2018. Effectiveness of a mindfulness-based social–emotional learning program on psychosocial adjustment and neuropsychological maturity in kindergarten children. *Mindfulness*, 10(1), pp.111–121.

Morris, M.C., Tangney, C.C., Wang, Y., Sacks, F.M., et al., 2015a. MIND diet slows cognitive decline with aging. *Alzheimer's & Dementia*, 11(9), pp.1015–1022.

Morris, M.C., Tangney, C.C., Wang, Y., Sacks, F.M., et al., 2015b. MIND diet associated with reduced incidence of Alzheimer's disease. *Alzheimer's & Dementia*, 11(9), pp.1007–1014.

Moszeik, E.N., von Oertzen, T., & Renner, K.-H., 2020. Effectiveness of a short yoga nidra meditation on stress, sleep, and well-being in a large and diverse sample. *Current Psychology*, 41, pp.5272–5286.

Munawar, K., Kuhn, S.K., & Haque, S., 2018. Understanding the reminiscence bump: a systematic review. *PLoS ONE*, 13(12), e0208595.

Naclerio, F., Seijo, M., Earnest, C.P., Puente-Fernández, P., & Larumbe-Zabala, E., 2020. Ingesting a post-workout vegan-protein multi-ingredient expedites recovery after resistance training in trained young males. *Journal of Dietary Supplements*, 18(6), pp.698–713.

Neumark-Sztainer, D., Watts, A.W., & Rydell, S., 2018. Yoga and body image: how do young adults practicing yoga describe its impact on their body image? *Body Image*, 27, pp.156–168.

Nidich, S.I., Rainforth, M.V., Haaga, D.A.F., Hagelin, J., et al., 2009. A randomized controlled trial on effects of the transcendental meditation program on blood pressure, psychological distress, and coping in young adults. *American Journal of Hypertension*, 22(12), pp.1326–1331.

Ong, J.C., Manber, R., Segal, Z., Xia, Y., Shapiro, S., & Wyatt, J.K., 2014. A randomized controlled trial of mindfulness meditation for chronic insomnia. *Sleep*, 37(9), pp.1553–1563.

Pandya, S.P., 2018. Yoga education program for improving memory in older adults: a multicity 5-year follow-up study. *Journal of Applied Gerontology*, 39(6), pp.576–587.

Parker, S., Bharati, S.V., & Fernandez, M., 2013. Defining yoga-nidra: traditional accounts, physiological research, and future directions. *International Journal of Yoga Therapy*, 23(1), pp.11–16.

Piitulainen, H., Seipäjärvi, S., Avela, J., Parvianinen, T., & Walker, S., 2018. Cortical proprioceptive processing is altered by aging. *Frontiers in Aging Neuroscience*, 10, p.147.

Prakash, R., Rastogi, P., Dubey, I., Abhishek, P., Chaudhury, S., & Small, B.J., 2012. Long-term concentrative meditation and cognitive performance among older adults. *Aging, Neuropsychology, and Cognition*, 19(4), pp.479–494.

Ramírez-Barrantes, R., Arancibia, M., Stojanova, J., Aspé-Sánchez, M., Córdova, C., & Henríquez, R.A., 2019. Default mode network, meditation, and age-associated brain changes: what can we learn from the impact of mental training on well-being as a psychotherapeutic approach? *Neural Plasticity*, 2019, pp.1–15.

Salem, G.J., Yu, S.S.-Y., Wang, M.-Y., Samarawickrame, S., et al., 2013. Physical demand profiles of Hatha yoga postures performed by older adults. *Evidence-Based Complementary and Alternative Medicine*, 2013, pp.1–29.

Seli, P., Beaty, R.E., Marty-Dugas, J., & Smilek, D., 2019. Depression, anxiety, and stress and the distinction between intentional and unintentional mind wandering. *Psychology of Consciousness: Theory, Research, and Practice*, 6(2), pp.163–170.

Sharpe, E., Lacombe, A., Butler, M.P., Hanes, D., & Bradley, R., 2020. A closer look at yoga nidra: sleep lab protocol. *International Journal of Yoga Therapy*, 31(1), Article 20.

Sorrells, S.F., Paredes, M.F., Cebrian-Silla, A., Sandoval, K., et al., 2018. Human hippocampal neurogenesis drops sharply in children to undetectable levels in adults. *Nature*, 555(7696), pp.377–381.

Steinberg, L., 2008. A social neuroscience perspective on adolescent risk-taking. *Developmental Review*, 28(1), pp.78–106.

Stickgold, R., 2005. Sleep-dependent memory consolidation. *Nature*, 437(7063), pp.1272–1278.

van Praag, H., 2005. Exercise enhances learning and hippocampal neurogenesis in aged mice. *Journal of Neuroscience*, 25(38), pp.8680–8685.

Villemure, C., Čeko, M., Cotton, V.A., & Bushnell, M.C., 2015. Neuroprotective effects of yoga practice: age-, experience-, and frequency-dependent plasticity. *Frontiers in Human Neuroscience*, 9, p.281.

Wahbeh, H., & Nelson, M., 2019. iRest meditation for older adults with depression symptoms: a pilot study. *International Journal of Yoga Therapy*, 29(1), pp.9–17.

Zhang, R., & Volkow, N.D., 2019. Brain default-mode network dysfunction in addiction. *NeuroImage*, 200, pp.313–331.

Ziegler, D.A., Simon, A.J., Gallen, C.L., Skinner, S., et al., 2019. Closed-loop digital meditation improves sustained attention in young adults. *Nature Human Behaviour*, 3(7), pp.746–757.

Glossary

Acetylcholine is involved in a variety of functions, including contracting muscles, arousal, attention, memory, learning and recall.

Addiction is a treatable, chronic medical disease involving complex interactions among brain circuits, genetics, the environment and an individual's life.

Alternate nostril breathing is a technique that relies on breathing through one nostril at a time using the fingers to open and close each side in an alternating fashion.

Alzheimer's disease is a progressive neurodegenerative disorder.

Amygdala plays a role in fear, anxiety, anger and processing emotional memories.

Anterior cingulate cortex integrates thoughts and feelings for emotional learning as well as monitors focus during activities like meditation.

Anxiety is characterized by persistent and excessive worrying, irrational fear and panic attacks.

Astrocytes are star-shaped cells that shuttle nutrients to neurons and aid in neuron-to-neuron communication.

Autonomic nervous system relays information about automatic or involuntary responses.

Basal ganglia are a group of neurons located deep within the brain that help control voluntary movement.

Biomarkers are measurable substances that are indicative of a biological state.

Blood–brain barrier is a filter between the brain's blood vessels and the brain tissue, and it protects the brain against bacteria, viruses and toxins that could cause a brain infection or damage while letting in important nutrients.

Brainstem regulates many important functions, such as breathing, heart rate, blood pressure, consciousness and sleep–wake cycles. It consists of three main sections called the midbrain, pons and medulla oblongata.

Case studies are in-depth analyses of a single person, group, or situation.

Causation occurs when one variable is directly related to or *causes* the second variable.

Central nervous system includes the brain and the spinal cord.

Cerebellum helps with coordination, the timing of movement, precision, movement correction as well as motor memory.

Chemoreceptors in the carotid arteries send signals to the medulla in the brainstem about the level of oxygen in the blood.

Chemosensation is the ability to sense chemicals in order to smell.

Chronic inflammation occurs when the body releases inflammatory cells even when it is not being attacked. It is a key component of chronic illness and stress-related diseases.

Chronic pain is pain that lasts more than three months, and it can affect relationships, quality of life and productivity.

Cohort studies are common in yoga and meditation research where the researcher tracks a group of participants longitudinally, over time, typically before and after an intervention.

Corpus callosum is the bridge between the two hemispheres of the brain.

Correlation is a measure of how strongly two variables are related, but one may not cause the other.

Corticobulbar tract sends information to the brainstem regarding movement of the head, neck and body.

Corticospinal tract carries signals from the brain to the spinal cord to relay information about movement of the body.

Deep breathing is a technique used to invite relaxation throughout the body.

Default mode network includes parts of the prefrontal cortex, cingulate cortex, temporal lobe and hippocampus. It is active when the brain is not engaged in a goal-oriented task.

Depression is a mood disorder that is characterized by feelings of despondency and dejection.

Diaphragmatic breathing, also known as belly breathing, is a technique that activates the diaphragm to draw air into the lungs.

Dopamine is the main neurotransmitter used in the reward system of the brain.

Dorsal attention network is involved in focused attention and becomes less active during mind wandering.

Electroencephalography (EEG) is a method for examining the brain that detects the brain's electrical activity of large groups of neurons.

Enteric nervous system oversees most of the digestive functions, such as movements of the gastrointestinal tract, regulating the secretion of digestive fluids and hormones, and it stimulates the immune system.

Ependymal cells produce cerebrospinal fluid.

Epithelial cells help keep invaders from getting into the brain's blood system.

External validity is the ability to generalize results from a study to a broader population outside of the study.

Focused-attention meditation requires a focus or concentration on a specific object or theme, such as the breath or a visualization, while disengaging from the wandering mind.

Frontal lobe is located at the front of the brain and is responsible for many important tasks, such as integrating information to allow for decision making.

Gamma-aminobutyric acid (GABA) is an inhibitory neurotransmitter and reduces the amount of communication between neurons in the brain.

Glutamate is the main excitatory neurotransmitter in the brain.

Golgi tendon organs sense information about muscle tension.

Gray matter contains mostly the cell bodies of neurons and their dendrites as well as glial cells and capillaries.

Gyrification is the pattern and degree of cortical folding of the brain or how wrinkly the brain's surface appears. It is likely a measure of how many neurons there are in the brain.

Hippocampus is responsible for declarative memory, which is the memory of facts and events.

Hypothalamic-pituitary-adrenal (HPA) axis is a stress pathway that becomes activated when the sympathetic nervous system is triggered. The HPA axis produces stress hormones, such as cortisol, that can damage the brain when released on a sustained basis.

Insula or insular cortex is responsible for self-awareness and self-reflection, as it senses the interior state of the body.

Internal validity is when the results from one group within the study can be generalized to another group within the study.

Interoception is the ability to sense the internal state of the body.

Joint receptors provide information about joint position.

Loving-kindness and compassion meditation centers on cultivating love, kindness and compassion towards others and oneself using a variety of mental techniques.

Mantra recitation meditation involves the repeated recitation of a sound, word or phrase either out loud or in one's head to promote focus and intention.

Mechanoreceptors are activated when the body touches an object.

Medulla contains control centers for vital functions, such as breathing, heart rate and blood pressure. This region is also involved in reflexes like swallowing and even sneezing.

Meissner's corpuscles are touch receptors that respond to soft touch and vibrations.

Merkel nerve endings are touch receptors that detect continuous pressure.

Microglia are the brain's immune cells, and they monitor the brain's environment for any intruders, such as bacteria and viruses.

Midbrain is the top portion of the brainstem and is involved with the control of movement, sleep, temperature regulation, vision and hearing.

Mindful breathing is a breathing technique that focuses the attention on the breath.

Motor cortex helps to plan, control and execute movements.

Motor homunculus is a topographic representation of the body parts involved in movement, mapped onto the relevant areas in the primary motor cortex.

Motor learning involves learning a new movement, which can then be stored as a motor memory, also known as muscle memory.

Motor memory is also known as muscle memory.

Motor neurons are specialized neurons that extend from the brain or spinal cord to individual muscle fibers of a muscle to provide instructions about which muscles to move and how to move them.

Multiple sclerosis (MS) is an autoimmune disease of the central nervous system (brain and spinal cord) where the immune system mistakenly attacks the protective myelin sheath around nerve fibers in the central nervous system.

Muscle spindles are proprioceptive receptors that detect changes in muscle length.

Neurogenesis is the process of creating new neurons. It is thought to only occur in the hippocampus.

Neuromuscular junction is where motor neurons transfer instructions to muscle fibers about movement.

Nociceptors are specialized neurons that detect thermal, physical and chemical pain.

Norepinephrine is used in the brain and body to prepare for arousal during exercise, stress and danger.

Occipital lobe is home to the main visual processing center, the primary visual cortex.

Oligodendrocytes help to insulate the axons of neurons in the brain that travel long distances by wrapping them in a protective myelin sheath.

Open monitoring meditation is where the attention is brought to the present moment without a focus on a specific object.

Osteoarthritis occurs when the cartilage between bones breaks down, damaging the joints.

Otolith organs sense forward and backward movements as well as gravity.

Pacinian corpuscles are sensitive touch receptors that respond to vibration.

Parasympathetic nervous system controls the relaxation response. It helps the body calm down, relax the muscles and digest food.

Parietal lobe processes sensory information, such as taste, touch, temperature, pain and pressure.

Peripheral nervous system consists of the neurons and nerves that stretch throughout the body.

Perspectives and editorials rely on someone's opinion instead of the data from a specific study.

Photoreceptors relay signals to the occipital lobe providing visual information.

Pons contains groups of neurons that are involved in sleep, respiration, equilibrium and many more functions.

Post-traumatic stress disorder (PTSD) is a trauma- or stress-related disorder that involves persistent mental and emotional stress, sleep disturbances and vivid recall of a stressful experience.

Pranayama is a group of techniques for breath control.

Prefrontal cortex is involved in cognitive control, decision making, attention and behavior.

Premotor cortex assists in the integration of sensory and movement information to prepare a movement.

Primary motor cortex is the main brain region involved in the control and execution of voluntary movements.

Proprioception is awareness of the position and movement of the body.

Purkinje cells are intricately branched neurons involved in the control of movement as well as learning.

Qualitative data is descriptive in nature and represented with language, instead of numbers.

Quantitative data refers to information that can be counted or measured.

Randomized control trials are where participants are randomly assigned to either the experimental group (the group receiving the intervention, i.e., practicing yoga or meditation) or the control group.

Reflex is a rapid, automatic movement that does not involve the brain.

Resilience is the ability to recover or "bounce back" after experiencing stress.

Resting-state networks are networks of brain regions that are active when the brain is not engaged in a specific activity or task.

Reviews combine evidence from multiple research studies.

Rheumatoid arthritis is a chronic inflammatory disorder affecting the joints.

Ruffini endings are touch receptors that respond when the skin is stretched and when there is an angle change in the joints.

Sample size is the population chosen for an experiment.

Schwann cells help to insulate nerves in the peripheral nervous system.

Sciatic nerve is the longest and largest nerve in the body.

Scientific evidence is derived from a well-controlled study that statistically either supports or counters a hypothesis or theory.

Semicircular canals detect rotational head movements: nodding up and down, shaking side to side and tilting left and right.

Sensory homunculus is a representation of the proportion of the somatosensory cortex that is devoted to each part of the body.

Sensory neuron is a nerve cell that detects and responds to the environment.

Serotonin helps regulate mood, sleep and appetite.

Somatic nervous system carries information about voluntary movement.

Somatomotor cortices are regions of the brain involved in processing tactile information, such as touch and pain.

Spinal cord is a bundle of nerves that extends about about 46 centimeters (18 inches) from the brain to the lumbar vertebrae in the lower back.

Statistical significance is a measure of confidence that two variables are related in some way and that the result is not due to chance.

Stress is a state of mental, emotional or physical strain resulting from adverse or demanding circumstances.

Stroke occurs when part of the brain stops receiving blood.

Supertasters are people who were born with more taste buds than the average person.

Supplementary motor area (SMA) plays a role in the control of movement, postural control and coordinating two-handed movements.

Sympathetic nervous system is activated during periods of stress as well as rigorous activity. It controls the fight, flight or freeze response when faced with danger.

Temporal lobe is involved in a variety of activities including hearing, listening, language, visual processing of faces and objects as well as memory.

Traumatic brain injury (TBI) is an injury to the head that causes damage to the brain.

Variables are people, places or things that scientists are trying to measure in some way.

Vestibular system helps the brain detect head movement and aids in gaze stability.

White matter appears white and contains mostly neuronal axons, which are the long cords that extend out from the cell body.

Yoga is a meditative movement practice derived from a spiritual practice from India.

Yoga nidra is a type of meditative yoga practice that can promote sleep and relaxation while decreasing stress and anxiety.

Subject Index

acetylcholine 29, 72
addiction 152–4
ADHD 161
adolescents 160–1
adrenocorticotrophic hormone (ACTH) 112
adults (yoga/meditation for) 163–4
ahimsa 172
alternate nostril breathing 89, 90–1
Alzheimer's disease
    and blood–brain barrier 142–3
    meditation for 143
    overview 141–3
    yoga for 143–4
amygdala 41, 124–5
amyloid beta protein 142
anterior cingulate cortex 45, 101–2, 122
anxiety
    causes of 120–1
    children/adolescents 161
    meditation for 121–2
    mindful breathing for 86–7
    yoga for 121
arthritis 149–51
astrocytes 31
auditory ossicles 53–4
autonomic nervous system 23

baby yoga 158–9
balance system 75–7
basal ganglia 70
biomarkers 114–5
blindness/visual impairment 50
blood oxygenation 85
blood–brain barrier 142–3
brain
    in adulthood 163–4
    aging brain 164–8

amygdala 41, 124–5
Broca's area 39
cerebellum 43, 71–2
    in childhood/adolescence 160
corpus callosum 42–3, 100–2
default mode network 107–8, 167–8
diet and 171–2
dorsal attention network 168
exercise and the 165
frontal lobe 36–9
glial cells 30–1, 42
gray matter 38–9, 41–2, 45–6, 100–4
gyrification 102–3
hemispheres of 41, 42–3
hippocampus 40–1, 102, 106–7, 124
in infancy 157
medulla 44–5, 84–5
midbrain 44
neurons 28
neurotransmitters 28–30
occipital lobe 43
overview 27–8, 36
parietal lobe 43
pons 44
prefrontal cortex 38, 101
resting-state networks 106–8
size of 42, 100
temporal lobe 39–43
Wernicke's area 39
white matter 38–9, 46, 100–2, 104
yoga as protective of 166
brainstem 44
breath/breathing
    alternate nostril breathing 89, 90–1
    blood oxygenation 85
    and the brain 84–7
    children/adolescents 162
    conscious control of 87–91

cultivating resilience with 91–2
deep breathing 88, 89–90
diaphragmatic breathing 89, 90
in free diving 88
human gas exchange 82
importance of the nose 83–4
mindful breathing 86–7, 88
and mood 85–7
nasal cycle 83–4
parabrachial nucleus and 86–7
physiology of 81–2
in Swara yoga 83
through stress 86–7
Broca's area 39

C-reactive protein (CRP) 115, 116
carotid artery 85
case studies 16
causation 18
cerebellum 43, 71–2
chair yoga 135–6, 139–40, 169–70
chakras 51
chanting 55–6
children
    ADHD 161
    benefits of yoga/meditation for 160
    mental health 160–2
    teaching yoga to 161
chocolate meditation 59–60
chronic inflammation 114–6
chronic pain 145–8
cingulate cortex 45–6, 101–2, 105–6
circadian rhythms 51, 173
clary sage oil 58
closed brain injury 131–2
cochlear implants 54
cognition (yoga and meditation for) 143–4, 166–7
cohort studies 16
complex regional pain syndrome (CRPS) 145
corpus callosum 42–3, 100–2
correlation 18–9
cortical thickness 38, 99–100
corticobulbar tract 69
corticospinal tract 69
corticotropin-releasing hormone (CRH) 112
cortisol 112–3
cranial nerves 60–1

deafness 54
deep breathing 88, 89–90
default mode network 107–8, 167–8
depression
    children/adolescents 161

meditation for 127–8
overview 124–5
yoga for 125–8
diaphragmatic breathing 89, 90
diet and brain health 171–2
DMT (N,N-dimethyltryptamine) 52
dopamine 29
dorsal attention network 168
dualism 91

early childhood (yoga in) 157–9
ears
    auditory ossicles 53–4
    and balance 75–7
Einstein, Albert 42
electroencephalography (EEG) 108–9
emotional pain 144–5
enteric nervous system 26–7
ependymal cells 31
epithelial cells 31
erectile tissue (in the nose) 83–4
essential oils 57–9
Essential Properties of Yoga Questionnaire 14–5
eucalyptus oil 58
exercise benefits 164–5
explicit memory 40–1

"fight, flight or freeze" response 112
focused-attention meditation 95–7, 104, 107
free diving 88
frontal lobe 36–9

Gage, Phineas 37
gamma-aminobutyric acid (GABA) 29
gaze stabilization 77
glial cells 30–1, 42
glutamate 29
golgi tendon organs 75
gray matter 38–9, 41–2, 45–6, 100–4
guided meditation 55
gustatory cortex 60–1
gut microbiome 27
gyrification 102–3

hands (brain area for) 68
headstands 135
hearing 53–6
hearing devices 54
hippocampus 40–1, 102, 106–7, 124
hypothalamic-pituitary-adrenal (HPA) axis 112, 123

immune system functioning 116-8
implicit memory 40-1
inclusivity 163
infants (yoga for) 157-9
inflammation 114-6
insular cortex 45-6, 100-1, 105
interleukin 115, 117
iRest 174

joint receptors 75

lavender oil 58, 59
limbic system 120-1
LoveYourBrain Yoga 133
loving-kindness meditation 46, 97, 105, 107
lower back pain 146-8

magnetoencephalography (MEG) 106
mandarin essential oil 59
mantra 55-6
mantra meditation 96-7, 105, 107-8
mechanoreceptors 62-4
meditation
    brain networks involved in 106-8, 167-8
    effect on brain function 104-9
    effect on brain structure 99-104
    focused-attention 95-7, 104, 107
    loving-kindness 46, 97, 105, 107
    mindfulness meditation 97-8
    movement regions of brain activated during 105
    open monitoring meditation 97-9, 105, 107
medulla 44-5, 84-5
Meissner's corpuscles 62
memory
    hippocampus and 40-1
    muscle 72
    smells and 57
Merkel nerve endings 62
microbiome 27
microglia 30
midbrain 44
MIND diet 171-2
mind-body connection 91-2
mindful breathing 86-7, 88
mindfulness meditation 97-8
motion sickness 77
motor cortex 67-9
motor homunculus 68
motor learning 72
movement
    basal ganglia and 70
    cerebellum and 71-2
    involuntary 74
    motor cortex 67-9
    motor learning 72
    motor neurons 72
    premotor cortex 69-70
    proprioception 74-9
    reflexes 74
    supplementary motor area 70
    voluntary 67-73
multiple sclerosis (MS)
    meditation for 141
    overview 137-8
    yoga for 138-40
muscle memory 72
muscle spindles 75
music therapy 54-5
myelin sheath 30, 38-9, 137-8

nasal cycle 83-4
nervous system
    autonomic nervous system 23
    enteric nervous system 26-7
    parasympathetic nervous system 23-4, 26, 85-6, 113-4
    somatic nervous system 23
    spinal cord 31-2
    sympathetic nervous system 23-4, 85-6, 112, 113
    vagus nerve 26, 85
networks
    default mode network 107-8, 167-8
    dorsal attention network 168
    resting-state networks 106-8
neurogenesis 165
neuromuscular junction 72
neurons 28
neuroplasticity 165
neurotransmitters 28-30
nicotine addiction 152-4, 153
nociceptors 144
norepinephrine 29, 123
nose (role in breathing) 83-4

occipital lobe 43
older adults 164-71
olfactory cortex 57
oligodendrocytes 30
open monitoring meditation 97-9, 105, 107
osteoarthritis 149
otolith organs 76-7

Pacinian corpuscles 62
pain
    and the brain 144–5
    chronic 145–8
    emotional pain 144–5
    lower back 146–8
    meditation for 146, 147
    mindful breathing and 86–7
    yoga for 146–8
parabrachial nucleus 86–7
parasympathetic nervous system 23–4, 26, 85–6, 113–4
parietal lobe 43
peppermint oil 58
personality change 37
photoreceptors 49–50
pineal gland 51–2
plant-based diets 171–2
pons 44
post-traumatic stress disorder (PTSD) 122–4
pranayama 87–8
pre-Bötzinger complex 85–6
prefrontal cortex 38, 101
premotor cortex 69–70
primary motor cortex 68–9
proprioception 74–9
prosopagnosia 39–40
Purkinje cells 71

qualitative data 17
quantitative data 17

randomized control trials 16
reflexes 74
relaxation response 91–2
research
    causation 18
    challenges in 15
    correlation 18–9
    methodologies/study design 15–6
    quantitative vs. qualitative methods 17
    sample size 17–8
    sections within published study 19
    validity 17
    variables 15
resilience (cultivating) 91–2, 118–20
resilience meditation 92, 119
resting-state networks 106–8
restorative yoga 24–5
reviews (in research) 16
rheumatoid arthritis 149
Richardson, Natasha 132

rosemary oil 58
Ruffini endings 62

safety for older yogis 168–70
sample size 17–8
Sanskrit effect 167
Schwann cells 31, 32
sciatic nerve 73
secondary brain injury 132
semicircular canals 75–7
senses meditation 64–5
sensory experience *see* hearing; sight; smell; taste; third eye; touch
sensory homunculus 63
serotonin 26, 29, 120
serotonin-reuptake inhibitors (SSRIs) 125
Shamatha meditation 96
sight
    blindness/visual impairment 50
    photoreceptors 49–50
singing bowls 55
sleep 173–4
smell
    chemosensation 56–7, 84–5
    essential oils 57–9
    and memory 57
    olfactory cortex 57
somatic nervous system 23
somatosensory cortex 62–3
sound baths 54–5
spinal cord 31–2
spine (yoga sequence for) 33
statistical significance 18
stress
    brain's stress system 112–3
    breathing through 86–7
    and chronic inflammation 114–6
    hormones 112–3, 123
    and immune system 116–8
    overview of 111–2
stroke
    meditation for 137
    overview 134
    yoga for 135–6
sun salutations 72
supertasters 61
supplementary motor area 70
Swara yoga 83
sympathetic nervous system 23–4, 85–6, 112, 113

taste 59–62
taste buds 60–1
tea tree oil 58, 59

telomerase 117
temporal lobe 39–43
third eye 51–3
tinnitus 54
touch
    filtering out signals 63
    mechanoreceptors 62–4
    sensory homunculus 63
    somatosensory cortex 62–3
trauma 118
traumatic brain injury (TBI)
    overview 131–3
    yoga/meditation for 133
treatment-induced addiction 152
tumor necrosis factor alpha (TNF-α) 115

vagus nerve 26, 85
validity 17
variables 15
vestibular system 75–7
Vipassana meditation 98
visual impairment 50

Wernicke's area 39
white matter 38–9, 46, 100–2, 104

yoga (definition) 14
yoga nidra 173–4

Zen meditation 98–9

Author Index

Abhang, P.A. 55
Acabchuk, R.L. 133
Afonso, R.F. 38
Ahmad, S. 27
Ahn, E.J. 16
Alden, S. 123
Aleman, A. 45
Alexiades, V. 49
Ali, B. 57, 58
Allen, N.J. 30
Alshaikh, J.T. 54
American Association of Neurological Surgeons (AANS) 131
American Society of Addiction Medicine (ASAM) 152
American Society of Anesthesiologists 145
Amin, A. 55
Anasuya, B. 24
Andel, R. 143
Annese, J. 40
Anxiety and Depression Association of America (ADAA) 120, 124
Apinhasmit, W. 31
Arain, M. 160
Asare, F. 27
Ates, G. 142
Averill, L.A. 123

Badlangana, N.L. 69
Bahney, J. 43
Balderson, B.H. 147
Band, G.P. 85
Bao, X. 57
Bardin, L. 29
Barnard, N. 171
Barres, B.A. 30
Bartoshuk, L. 61
Beauchemin, J. 160

Benson, H. 91
Berendsen, A.M. 172
Berger, M. 26
Bernier, R. 55
Berridge, C.W. 29
Berryhill, M. 43
Bharati, S.V. 174
Bhargav, H. 91
Bhasin, M.K. 116
Bhattacharyya, K.K. 143
Bhavanani, A.B. 90
Black, D.S. 162
Blanck, P. 121
Blumenrath, S. 62, 63, 144
Bock, B.C. 154
Bondarenko, E.A. 124, 125
Boonpirak, N. 31
Bormann, J.E. 55
Bowden, D.E. 101
Braboszcz, C. 109
Brain from Top to Bottom, The 69
Brand, M. 24
Brandmeyer, T. 95, 97, 108, 166
Braun, K.L. 123
Brenes, G.A. 143
Brewer, J. 107, 153
Bridges, L. 124, 125
Brinkman, C. 70
Brosel, S. 168
Brough, D. 115
Buchanan, A. 121
Buchanan, T.W. 116
Bushdid, C. 57
Bushnell, M.C. 144, 145
Butzer, B. 160

Cahn, B.R. 109

187

Camilleri, M. 26
Cao, J. 173
Carlson, L.E. 98
Carpenter, L.L. 123
Carson, C.F. 58
Cascella, M. 73
Cavalera, C. 141
Cejudo, J. 162
Cekic, M. 98
Ceko, M. 144, 145
Centers for Disease Control and Prevention (CDC) 14, 134, 149, 164
Cerrillo-Urbina, A.J. 161
Chambers, D.A. 17
Chang, R.B. 85
Chayer, C. 37
Chen, Y. 168
Cherkin, D.C. 147
Cherup, N.P. 75, 78
Chiesa, A. 98
Ching, H.-H. 160
Chow, T.W. 37
Clark, R.E. 39, 40
Clarke, T.C. 14
Coles, J.A. 30
Collette-Merrill, K. 174
Collings, V.B. 60
Conner, J.M. 63
Corey, J.P. 83
Costandi, M. 42, 100
Courtiol, E. 57
Coutinho, J.F. 168
Coyle, J.T. 29
Cramer, H. 121
Cressman, V.L. 160
Crisan, M. 51, 52
Critchley, H.D. 46
Crocker, J. 144
Crow, E.M. 32
Curtis, S. 54
Cushing, R.E. 123

Dahlhamer, J. 145
Damasio, A. 91
Danhauer, S.C. 24
Darragh, A.R. 121
De Gennaro, L. 173
de Kloet, C.S. 123
Deepak, K.K. 24
Delorme, A. 95, 97, 108, 109, 166
DeMartini, C. 55
Devaney, K. 168
Devinsky, O. 45

Devlin, K. 54
Devore, E.E. 172
Dijkstra, B.W. 70
Dinenno, F.A. 113
Ditre, J.W. 152
Ditto, B. 163
Djalilova, D.M. 115
Dol, K.S. 173, 174
Doll, A. 86
Donahoe-Fillmore, B. 160
Donnelly, K.Z. 133
Donoghue, J.P. 68
Dudai, Y. 61
Dunlop, B.W. 123
Dunne, J.D. 98
Dutheil, F. 89

Eclache, M. 163
Eichenbaum, H. 39, 40
Eisenbeck, N. 89
Eising, C. 117
El-Sohemy, A. 61
Elangovan, N. 78
Emavardhana, T. 98
Epel, E.S. 117
Erickson, K.I. 165
Eriksson, P.S. 165
Erkkilä, J. 54
España, R.A. 29
Evans, S. 149
Eyre, H.A. 167

Faber, J. 17
Falcone, G. 89
Falkenberg, R.I. 117
Falsafi, N. 127
Fang, C.Y. 116
Feng, J. 59
Fernandez, M. 174
Fernando, R. 162
Ferreira-Vorkapic, C. 174
Filler, A.G. 73
Fine, E.J. 71
Fleming, M.A. 26, 27
Fonseca, L.M. 17
Fournier, D. 133
Fox, K.C.R. 96, 100, 101, 102, 104, 105
Franjic, D. 165
Freedman, M. 37
Freeman, J.R. 13
Freund, H.-J. 69
Friedman, A. 142

Gage, F.H. 104, 165
Gao, W. 157
Garcia-Larrea, L. 43
Gard, T. 163
Garland, S.N. 98
Garrett, R. 135
Garrison, K.A. 107, 108, 168
Gawali, B.W. 55
George, T. 152
Geretsegger, M. 54
Gerritsen, R.J. 85
Gershon, M.D. 27
Gheban, B.A. 51, 52
Gilmore, J.H. 157
Glasgow, R.E. 17
Goddard, A.W. 29
Goff, D.C. 29
Goldberg, S. 127, 133
Goldin, P.R. 98
Goldman, N. 163
Golshan, S. 84
Gómez Gallego, M. 54
Gómez García, J. 54
Gorgoni, M. 173
Gosain, A. 114
Gothe, N.P. 41, 166, 167
Gotink, R.A. 41
Goyal, M. 113
Grabara, M. 32
Grant, E. 160
Gray, J.A. 26
Groessl, E.J. 15, 147
Gross, J.J. 98
Gross, T. 84
Grossman, P. 46
Gruzelier, J. 101
Gunjawate, D.R. 54

Hagen, I. 161
Hamilton, J. 87
Hansen, D.V. 30
Hanson, J.E. 30
Haque, S. 160
Harrington, A. 98
Hartzell, J.F. 167
Harvard Health Publishing 124
Harvard University 157
Hashimoto, K. 44
Hauber, W. 70
Hawkins, J. 27
Hearon, C.M. 113
Heather, S. 54, 55
Heck, D.H. 89

Hellhammer, D.H. 117
Henley, D.V. 59
Herculano-Houzel, S. 27, 42, 43
Hillier, S. 135
Hilton, L. 101, 123, 145
Hodgkin, A.L. 31
Hoge, E.A. 121, 122
Honk, J. 70
Hoolahan, J. 121
Horton, J. 173
Huang, Z. 165
Hummelsheim, H. 69
Hunt, T. 55
Hutchins, T.L. 160
Huxley, A.F. 31

Idriss, H.T. 115
Ikeda, K. 84, 157
Immink, M.A. 135
Innes, K.E. 149
Ionita, C.C. 71
iRest 174

Jacob, M.H. 30
Jain, R. 51
James-Palmer, A. 161
Jarraya, S. 160
Jaryal, A. 24
Jeannot, E. 32
Jerram, M. 89
Jia, W. 27
Jiang, C.-L. 112, 114
Johns Hopkins Medicine 132, 133
Johnson, E.O. 75
Johnson, R.L. 26

Kahana-Zweig, R. 83, 84
Kalaivani, S. 90
Kalueff, A.V. 29
Kamath, A. 90
Kanaya, A.M. 24
Kang, H. 16
Kaplan, R.M. 17
Karnath, H.O. 43
Katz, B. 31
Kemper, K.J. 91
Kempermann, G. 104
Kennedy, D. 58
Kenny, M. 55
Khalsa, D.S. 55
Khalsa, S.B. 160
Khanal, H. 49

Khirallah, M. 91
Kiecolt-Glaser, J.K. 115
Kim, D.-Y. 26
Kim, H. 172
Kirschbaum, C. 117
Kishimoto, T. 115
Klaassens, E.R. 123
Knecht, S. 39
Knickmeyer, R.C. 157
Kolasinski, S.L. 149
Kosten, T. 152
Koulouris, A. 149
Kovar, K. 58
Kraftl, P. 173
Kramer, A.F. 166, 167
Kross, E. 145
Kuhn, S.K. 160
Kumari, M.J. 90
Kunkle, B.W. 142
Kuo, Y.-M. 165
Kurth, F. 103
Kwon, D. 71

Lammens, R. 70
Lardone, A. 106, 107
Larkin, M. 137
Lauche, R. 149
Lawrence, M. 135
Lazar, S.W. 99
Leak, R.K. 51
Leckie, R.L. 165
Lee, H.K. 158
Lemay, V. 121
Leong, H. 24
Leppla, L. 54
Lerch, J.P. 38
Levin, A.B. 141
Lin, T.-W. 165
Liu, S. 86, 152
Liu, X. 101
Liu, Y.-Z. 112, 114
Livingston, E. 174
Lohr, L. 71
Lopez-Castejon, G. 115
Low, L.A. 144, 145
Lu, P. 32
Luan, Y.Y. 115
Luciano, C. 89
Luders, E. 102, 103
Lupien, S.J. 112
Lutz, A. 13

Ma, X. 90
McAuley, E. 166, 167
McCall, C.M. 26
MacDonald, C. 158
McLennan, D. 101
Madanmohan 90
Magnon, V. 89
Malik, S.S. 88
Mallya, A.P. 160
Malouff, J.M. 117, 118
Malpaux, B. 51
Manandhar, S.A. 90
Manassero, C.A. 59
Martin, E.I. 120, 122
Martinez, N. 55
Matiz, A. 119
Matthews, P.B. 75
Mauguière, F. 43
Mayo Clinic 32
Mehrotra, S.C. 55
Mehta, S. 161
Meiri, N. 61
Melville, G.W. 55
Minai, M. 71
Minvaleev, R.S. 135
Mischkowski, D. 144
Modinos, G. 45
Mohanty, S. 50, 75
Moore, R.Y. 51, 52
Moran, S. 96
Moreno-Gómez, A.-J. 162
Morrell, M.J. 45
Morris, M.C. 172
Moszeik, E.N. 173
Munawar, K. 160
Muzio, M.R. 73

Naclerio, F. 172
Nagathna, R. 75
Nagel, S.J. 31
Naismith, J.H. 115
Narazaki, M. 115
National Center for Complementary and Integrative Health (NCCIH) 14
National Institute of Environmental Health Services (NIEHS) 59
National Multiple Sclerosis Society 138
Naveen, K.V. 83
Nayar, U.S. 161
Nelson, M. 174
Nestor, J. 84, 90
Neumark-Sztainer, D. 163
Newman, E.A. 31

Ng, B.A. 83
Nichols, D.E. 51, 52
Nidich, S.I. 163
Nuckowska, M.K. 88
Nutt, D.J. 29

Olson, I.R. 43
Omkar, S.N. 32
Ong, J.C. 173
Ormel, J. 45
Owens, L.R. 96

Pace, T.W.W. 116
Pagnoni, G. 98
Pal, G.K. 90
Pande, S. 55
Pandya, S.P. 166
Pantelyat, A. 54
Parhi, K.K. 27
Park, C.L. 14
Parker, S. 174
Patterson, F. 160
Perry, G. 55, 56
Peters, M.L. 117
Phillips, K.A. 42
Piitulainen, H. 168
Pirke, K.-M. 117
Polich, J. 109
Polito, V. 56
Posadzki, P. 152
Posner, M.I. 45
Prabhakar, N.R. 84
Pradhan, B. 75
Prajapati, R. 90
Prakash, R. 166
Pramanik, T. 90
Preuschoff, K. 46
Proctor, W. 91
Pudasaini, B. 90

Qaseem, A. 146

Rai, R.K. 83
Rain, M. 87
Ramírez-Barrantes, R. 168
Ramsey, R.G. 83
Ranganath, C. 39, 40
Rankhambe, H. 55
Rao, M. 27
Ravi, R. 54
Reangsing, C. 127
Reber, P.J. 41

Renner, K.-H. 173
Richter-Levin, G. 118
Rieder, R. 27
Rittiwong, T. 127
Rolls, E. 57
Rosca, I.A. 51, 52
Rosenblum, K. 61
Rosenkranz, M.A. 117
Rosenzweig, S. 98
Roth, B.L. 26
Rydell, S. 163

Sacks, O. 39
Salem, G.J. 171
Sandi, C. 118
Sanes, J.N. 68
Sanjay, Z. 90
Santamaría, A.J. 32
Sarapas, C. 123
Saraswati, S.M. 83
Saritas, E.U. 31
Schmeichel, B.E. 29
Schneider, J.K. 127
Schöne, B. 89
Schutte, N.S. 117, 118
Schwartz, A.B. 67
Sciarrino, N.A. 123
Segura-Aguilar, J. 29
Seijo-Martinez, M. 44
Seli, P. 168
Senatorov, V.V. 142
Shadrina, M. 124, 125
Shannahoff-Khalsa, D. 84
Sharma, A. 145
Sharma, M. 124, 125
Sharpe, E. 173
Sheline, Y.I. 124
Sheng, M. 30
Shenoy, A.K. 90
Sherman, K.J. 147
Shin, L.M. 122
Shulman, R. 56
Si, B. 29
Simon, R. 108
Simpson, F.M. 55, 56
Simrén, M. 27
Singer, T. 46
Singh, K. 91
Singh, S.P. 106
Siponkoski, S.T. 54
Slominsky, P.A. 124, 125
Smale, G. 100
Small, B.J. 143

Solakoglu, O. 78
Song, E. 29
Song, H. 104
Sorrells, S.F. 165
Southwick, S.M. 123
Spampinato, C. 59
Speh, J.C. 51
Squire, L.R. 39, 40
Srinivasan, T.M. 91
Starcke, K. 24
Stark, C.E.L. 39, 40
Steinberg, L. 160
Stickgold, R. 173
Stone, L.M. 60
Störsrud, S. 27
Strauss, C. 145
Streeter, C.C. 26, 125
Strupp, M. 168
Stump, E. 132
Sun, L.-N. 123
Szopa, J. 32

Tanaka T. 115
Tang, Y.-Y. 45
Tassadaq, N. 88
Tavassoli, S. 27
Teasdale, H. 157
Telles, S. 24, 83
Temburni, M.K. 30
Tetzlaff, K. 88
Thayabaranathan, T. 135
Thompson, W. 55, 56
Tilbrook, H.E. 146
Tori, C.D. 98
Trewhela, A. 32
Tsai, S.-F. 165

Unnikrishnan, N.K. 27
Urval, R.P. 90

Valdivia-Salas, S. 89
Vallet, G.T. 89
Van Aalst, J. 14, 41
Van Dam, N.T. 46
van Eijndhoven, P. 125
van Kordelaar, J. 77

van Praag, H. 165
Vempati, R.P. 24
Venkatesh, H.N. 114
Verwey, W.B. 70
Vestergaard-Poulsen, P. 44
Vigen, T. 18
Villemure, C. 43, 45, 166
Vishwas, S. 32
Vogt, B.A. 45
Volkow, N.D. 168
Vollbehr, N.K. 121
Von Bartheld, C.S. 43
von Oertzen, T. 173

Wahbeh, H. 95, 97, 108, 166, 174
Walia, N. 152
Wang, Y.-X. 112, 114
Wathugala, M. 137
Watkins, L.E. 123
Watts, A.W. 163
Way, B.M. 144
Weaver, I.J. 121
Weinstein, A.M. 165
Wells, R.E. 143
Wieland, L.S. 146
Wilkins, R.W. 54
Wilson, C.G. 26
Wilson, D.A. 57
Wolkowitz, O.M. 117
Wong, A. 123
World Health Organization 153

Xue, S. 45

Yackle, K. 85
Yao, Y.M. 115
Yoga Journal 72
Yonelinas, A.P. 39, 40
Yong, E. 56

Zaccaro, A. 89
Zhang, J. 168
Zhang, R. 168
Zhang, Y. 14
Ziegler, D.A. 163

'With ease, experience and tons of research, Fair swiftly weaves connections between the relatively new practice of neuroscience and the centuries-long practices of yoga and meditation."
—**Ashley Juavinett**, PhD, author of *So You Want to Be a Neuroscientist?*

'In an easily digestible format, *The Neuroscience of Yoga and Meditation* is a one-of-a-kind resource that provides yoga teachers tools to create deeply impactful classes for students."
—**Caitlin Pascucci**, E-RYT500, Founder of Sangha Studio

'As an occupational therapist, I look forward to referencing this text when I use movement and breathwork with my clients. I particularly appreciate the inclusivity of different physical conditions to support the broad population I serve in the disability community."
—**Sharon Bergmann, OTR/L**

The Neuroscience of Yoga and Meditation presents a comprehensive review of scientific research on the effects of yoga and meditation on the brain. The author offers tools for interpreting scientific literature and explores the current limitations in studying these practices. She also includes examples of meditations and movement routines that activate the brain to decrease stress and improve well-being.

The Neuroscience of Yoga and Meditation is a must-have for any yoga teacher, yoga therapist or yoga student who is interested in how contemplative practices affect the brain. Topics include:

- Anatomy of the brain
- How the senses work
- Movement and proprioception
- Breathing science
- Styles of meditation
- Stress, inflammation and trauma
- Psychological disorders and neurological conditions
- Brain plasticity and aging

Brittany Fair, MS, RYT200, RCYT is a San Diego-based science writer, podcast host and yoga teacher. With a background in philosophy, ecology, medical studies and neuroscience, she has taught courses and workshops at yoga studios, schools and universities nationwide. She is also the former president of the San Diego Science Writers Association. Outside of work, she is a competitive triathlete and twin mom.

Cover design by Bruce Hogarth

HANDSPRING PUBLISHING

ISBN 978-1-913426-43-9

www.handspring.com

@HandspringBooks